BACK TO LIFE
A Bladder Cancer Journey

BACK TO LIFE
A Bladder Cancer Journey

FRANK SADOWSKI

Foreword by Sia Daneshmand, M.D.

Cardboard Box Books
ISBN-13: 978-0692401217

Book design by Maureen Cutajar
www.gopublished.com

For Laura Ann Sadowski

Contents

Foreword

Metastatic bladder cancer is virtually incurable, with median survival rates measured in single-digit months. Most people are surprised to hear that bladder cancer is the 3rd most common cancer in men in the United States after lung cancer and prostate cancer, with 11,500 men estimated to die from the disease in 2015 (American Cancer Society: Cancer Facts and Figures 2015. Atlanta, GA). The best chance for cure is diagnosing the cancer early while it is confined to the bladder wall without spread to the lymph nodes or distant organs. Bladder cancer, like most other cancers, is staged using the TNM system where T denotes the depth of invasion within the bladder wall, N denotes the involvement of lymph nodes, and M denotes whether the cancer has spread to other organs. Low-grade bladder tumors generally are limited to the inner layer of the bladder, and do not invade the wall, whereas high-grade tumors have the ability and tendency to invade the deeper layers of the bladder, eventually leading to lymph node involvement and distant metastasis. Even high-grade Stage I bladder cancer (T1 in the TNM nomenclature), where the tumor has penetrated the lining between the inner surface of the bladder and the deeper muscle layer, is a potentially lethal disease that requires meticulous attention. Recognition of the critical nuances of early-stage bladder cancer can make the difference between life and death.

The high-grade T1 group represents about 20% of the patients who present with non-muscle-invasive bladder cancer. These tumors have a high propensity to recur and progress to muscle invasion with the associated risk of metastasis and death. Long-term studies show rates of progression to muscle invasion as high as 50% with more than 30% of patients eventually dying of bladder cancer. Although there is a refined understanding of some of the molecular mechanisms and biology of bladder cancer, the currently available medical armamentarium cannot adequately differentiate patients who are best suited for conservative management versus those who are destined to progress to metastatic disease.

Radical cystectomy (surgery to remove the bladder, surrounding lymph nodes, and in men, the prostate) provides the best chance for cure; however such surgery is associated with significant morbidities, including effects on urinary continence and on sexual and gastrointestinal function. Early cystectomy performed for high-grade T1 cancer generally allows for construction of a neobladder (a new bladder made from the patient's own small intestine) in most patients, and nerve-sparing approaches employed for preservation of sexual function. Even early radical cystectomy for high-grade T1 disease does not guarantee cure, indicating that a subset of these cancers has aggressive biologic behavior. The crux of the issue is balancing quality of life with effective cancer management.

Optimal outcomes can only be achieved by understanding the nuances of tumor biology, and by having a surgeon who interweaves his or her knowledge and experience with the patient's wishes to ensure preservation of *quality* as well as *quantity* of life. As a cancer surgeon, I derive the greatest satisfaction from seeing patients lead vibrant lives following treatment of a deadly cancer.

In this book Frank Sadowski recounts his poignant journey through diagnosis, decision-making, surgery, and the post-operative sequelae of undergoing a radical cystectomy. After accepting his diagnosis, Frank approaches his cancer treatment with resilience and determination. He learns about the *"two distinct and opposed schools of thought regarding treatment"* for his high-grade T1 diagnosis. His story is an intimate account of the quandary patients face when given choices regarding their cancer treatment. In the case of high-grade T1 bladder cancer, there are two vastly different management pathways. One is a conservative route, treating with medicine instilled in the bladder in the hopes of controlling the disease and preserving the organ. The other is a more radical approach involving extensive surgery to remove the bladder, prostate, and dozens of pelvic lymph nodes in an attempt to eradicate the disease at its roots, and provide the best chance at a durable cure.

This is the first book of its kind. There is a paucity of public attention to this prevalent disease, and bladder cancer research is severely underfunded. *Back to Life: A Bladder Cancer Journey* highlights this important subject and encourages patients and physicians alike to understand the dilemma from the patient's perspective and to appreciate the anguish they go through following the initial consultation. It is important to know that patients can fully emerge from the initial difficult recovery period following a radical cystectomy to lead unrestricted, productive lives. Through this honest and moving account of his cancer journey, Frank shows us how this can be done. His story should prove enlightening and inspiring to patients grappling with illness and difficult treatment decisions, as well as to medical professionals and indeed to anyone with an interest in how persons facing profound challenges find it within themselves to cope wisely and courageously.

Sia Daneshmand, M. D.
February 2015

Prologue

I knew even before I opened my eyes. I knew I was waking up from anesthesia. I knew I had undergone major surgery for bladder cancer. I knew I was in intensive care. And I was alive.

It was around 4 p.m. on Friday, December 21st, 2007, when these thoughts rose up in my consciousness from a deep black void. To my surprise, I was in no great hurry to open my eyes. I tried to move my leg as a kind of experiment, but I felt nothing. Tried the same with a hand and distinctly felt my fingers moving. OK, so it's time, I thought.

I opened my eyes. The first thing I saw was the smiling face of Dr. Sia Daneshmand, my surgeon. I croaked out a hello, realizing that my scratchy throat was probably due to having a pipe stuck down it for ... how long? More of the room came into focus and I saw my wife Laura standing behind my doctor.

"How did I do?" I asked. I realized Dr. Daneshmand had a hand on my shoulder.

"You did just fine," he said. "Just fine." I knew there was something else, something really important, that I was supposed to be asking him, but it wouldn't come. I passed out.

I have no idea if I was asleep for thirty seconds or thirty minutes, but I slowly came back to consciousness. When I opened my eyes Dr. Daneshmand was still there, as was Laura. Then all of a sudden everything came back to me in a rush. The cancer diagnosis. The TURBT. The decision. The operating room. And signing the last bit of paperwork, selecting my order of preference for urinary diversion after they took out my bladder. I remembered that this was necessary because the surgeon would not know exactly what was possible until he got in there. My choices had been: first, neobladder; second, internal pouch with stoma; and third, external bag with stoma. And suddenly the question I couldn't remember before was crystal clear, and hovered like a living, breathing presence between me, practically comatose in a hospital bed, and Dr. Daneshmand, nattily attired in scrubs over his dress shirt and slacks. I tried to lift my head to speak, but my neck muscles didn't answer my brain's command, so I just spoke from the pillow.

"What did I get?"

"You got the neobladder. Everything went perfectly. You did just fine."

I think I smiled. I know I tried to. I might have even said thank you. I know I tried to.

Then I passed out for a long time.

BLOOD

Chapter One

My bladder cancer experience began on Tuesday, October 30th, 2007. I had started a new job after leaving my position at Amazon.com in 2006. It required extensive travel, including spending two weeks of every month in a company apartment near the headquarters in Mahwah, New Jersey; one week in either Europe or Asia; and one week working from my home in Sammamish, Washington, just east of Seattle. It was my week at home and I had scheduled my annual physical for late that morning with my primary care physician. After the doctor, I headed to our health club located close by for a long workout, including two hours on the spinning cycle.

I headed home after a hot shower and started preparing dinner, drinking glass after glass of water due to the dehydrating effect of the hard aerobic exercise. Naturally, thirty minutes later I felt the strong urge to urinate. I asked my wife to watch the pot and headed into the hall bathroom to relieve myself.

But nothing happened. I couldn't pee! I took stock of the situation as a little tickle of fear ran up my spine. So I stood over the toilet and pushed hard. Splat! A large splash of bright red blood sprayed the toilet. But I still couldn't pee. Clearly, something was amiss. I cleaned the toilet, flushed, and calmly walked back into the kitchen.

"Turn off the stove," I said. "We're taking a little ride down to the emergency room." The town next to us, Issaquah, was just down the hill from the Sammamish plateau where we lived. It took about ten very uncomfortable minutes to get there, and as soon as I explained the problem I was whisked into an exam room. I felt as if I were going to explode at this point, so even though I had never been catheterized and was scared to death of it, I was quite willing if it would give me some relief. As a nurse scrubbed me up and prepared the catheter, the doctor was very calm and reassuring. He told me that I had probably gotten severely dehydrated and that a little blood from the vigorous cycling exercise had probably coagulated and blocked the urethra. In went the catheter, and I heard liquid splashing into the bucket, which I could not see. The nurse audibly sucked in a deep breath. My wife Laura was sitting next to me, and her face drained of color in seconds.

"Ah," said the doctor. "This is not so good."

All I felt was huge relief as the pressure relaxed. It was not painful.

"What?" I said.

"It's blood," he said. "Quite a lot of blood." He turned to the nurse and told her to measure the quantity as soon as I was drained, which took only about thirty seconds. As it turned out, they had drained 590 cc's of blood and urine from my bladder, more than a half liter. He told me they were going to prep me for an immediate CT scan.

The results of the scan were back in minutes. There was a large mass near the right ureter inside of my bladder. I asked what that meant, and he said that he couldn't say for sure, not being a urologist, but for sure it was not good. He told me they were putting me in an ambulance and taking me to the Swedish Medical Center hospital on First Hill in downtown Seattle. I would be admitted, spend the night and see the on-call urologist first thing the following morning. Laura drove behind the ambulance and made sure I got checked in and situated, then she left me and returned to our children.

Chapter Two

After a very restless night and a breakfast of cold scrambled eggs and lukewarm coffee, the urologist on duty walked in at 6:15 a.m. He was Dr. James Porter, and just by the luck of the draw he happened to be on call. This was the first of several chance occurrences that were to be incredibly important to my survival, but of course I had no way of knowing that. I smiled and joked about getting clogged up and the trip to the hospital in an ambulance, but he never cracked the slightest smile. Instead, he told me directly that he had viewed the CT scan results and felt there was almost a 100% chance that I had bladder cancer, due to the size and position of the mass. He told me he had seen this kind of result hundreds of times throughout his career, and he had never had a case that turned out *not* to be cancer. I asked what we could do to get it out of me and go on with my life. He gave me a stern look and asked me what I knew about bladder cancer. I told him I knew nothing, but that I was pretty fluent in cancer, having been a regional mentor for the Lance Armstrong Foundation for four years and the husband of a cancer survivor. He was unimpressed. He told me that what I had was extremely serious. He was careful to say he could not render a true diagnosis until he took the tumor out and tested it, but he was relatively sure I had a T3 Grade III bladder tumor. He unsmilingly suggested that I look it up on the Internet when I got home. I told him I would, but that I was scheduled to fly to Amsterdam that coming Sunday afternoon. He was, again, not amused.

"This is one of the most dangerous and fastest growing of all cancers, and is frequently fatal," he said. "You are not going anywhere for quite a while."

That got rid of the smiles and light conversation in a big hurry, let me tell you. I asked him when he wanted to take the tumor out and what the procedure entailed. He told me that due to the large amount of blood involved he needed to get me off the blood-thinning prescription-strength ibuprofen I was taking for an unrelated pain issue. He explained that the procedure, called a TURBT (transurethral resection of a bladder tumor) was performed under full anesthesia, and involved inserting a large catheter into the bladder and then putting a camera and a heated cutting device in through the catheter to cut out and cauterize the tumor site. It was Wednesday morning, October 31st. Dr. Porter scheduled the procedure for Friday morning, November 2nd, at his clinic, the Swedish Urology Group, just a few blocks from the hospital.

TURBT

Chapter Three

My wife picked me up that afternoon, and I related my conversation with Dr. Porter. As soon as I arrived home, I went to my second-floor office and booted up my work PC. The first sites I looked at contained general information about bladder cancer, but I quickly found a site that detailed the different tumor types and grades. Bladder tumors are typed from T0 through T3, and graded I through III by speed of growth. A T0 tumor means that the tumor is cancerous but is free-floating at the mucous-covered bladder wall, not yet growing into the wall. A T1 tumor is one that is growing into the mucous membrane but not yet invading the muscle wall. T2 indicates that the tumor is muscle-invasive but still contained within the bladder. T3 is when the cancer has broken through the outer muscle wall and is on the loose. The treatment for T2 and T3 bladder cancer is immediate surgery to remove the entire bladder, called a radical cystectomy. It was then I recalled Dr. Porter telling me he strongly suspected he was looking at a high-grade T3 tumor. The next page talked about survival rates, and chilled me to the bone. I had to read it three times, and realized I had never been more scared in my life.

The three-year survival rate for T3 bladder cancer is 5%.

I walked downstairs in a trance, and found Laura in the kitchen. She must have just walked in, as it was dusk outside and she had not yet turned a light on. She smiled and asked me what I had found out on line. "It's really, really bad," I said, "and if Dr. Porter is right I'm almost certainly going to die." We wrapped our arms around each other in the darkening kitchen. And then we cried.

Over the next two days I read everything I could get my hands on about bladder cancer. The more I learned the worse it looked. But my years of volunteer work with the Lance Armstrong Foundation served me very well. I looked at conventional and alternative treatments, digested reams of statistics on recurrence rates and survival chances, and also investigated Dr. Porter. As it turns out, I had been very lucky that he was on call that first morning. Not that Swedish Medical would have had anyone substandard, but Dr. Porter was the urological equivalent of a rock star, having been the head of urology at the University of Washington's teaching hospital for fifteen years prior to joining the Swedish Urology Group. So it appeared I was in very good hands, while at the same time lending additional, albeit unwanted, credibility to his preliminary opinion. I tried to focus on what he had first said, that we wouldn't know anything for certain about tumor type or grade until the post-TURBT pathology was completed.

I also learned that bladder cancer is largely a disease of older males, men being three times as likely as women to be diagnosed. At fifty-four, I was definitely on the younger side, as the average age of diagnosis in men is seventy-five!

At this point I contacted my primary care physician and gave her the full story to date. She was in disbelief that I could have had a full physical, including a complete urinalysis which showed not even microscopic amounts of blood, and yet have had the bleeding incident just a few short hours later. She even checked the "chain of custody" of my samples and had them retested, with the same negative results. I have asked each of the doctors I've been involved with about this, and it is a total mystery to all of them. It remains so to this day.

I checked in at the Swedish Urology Group in downtown Seattle a little after 6:00 a.m. on Friday, November 2nd. They started an IV, and after a half-hour wait Dr. Porter came in. As I was coming to realize, this guy is all business. He explained the procedure in great detail, pausing frequently to see if either Laura or I had questions, and assured me that the procedure was not dangerous. A few minutes later I was wheeled into the small operating room and introduced to the anesthesiologist. A goodbye to my wife and a weak smile later, out I went.

Chapter Four

I woke up less than an hour later, and the first thing I felt was the catheter. They had told me it would still be in place when I woke up, so I was not surprised. They had also told me that it was large in diameter, and they weren't kidding. I was in a small recovery room, and my wife was sitting across from me. She summoned a nurse, who came in and checked on me and told me Dr. Porter would be along soon. A few minutes later "Mr. Serious" came in and asked how I was feeling. I told him I was fine other than the discomfort from the catheter. He checked the collection bag and was glad to see almost no blood. He told me the procedure went fine and that I would be going home in an hour or so. I was to wait in recovery for a bit, then have the catheter removed. He told me that they would wait for me to be able to successfully pass a few blood-free cc's of urine, and after I that I was free to go.

So after another forty-five minutes and several checks from the nurse, I was led into another room to get the catheter out. Before walking into the procedure room, Dr. Porter said they had visiting nursing students from the University of Washington that day, and would I mind if a couple of them observed. I said sure. So here I was, my ass hanging out of that ridiculous backless "gown" and a pipe running down my leg to a bag. A pitiful old geezer, to say the least. The nurse came in, followed by Dr. Porter and two eighteen- or nineteen-year-old female students. They told me to take off the gown, and Dr. Porter said the nurse would remove the catheter slowly so as not to cause any damage. He also said I might experience some "mild discomfort" as it was removed. If you've been around doctors or hospitals at all, you already know that when a doctor says you may experience mild discomfort he is really saying this will hurt more than anything in your life thus far. He did not disappoint. Picture me standing naked in a freezing cold room in front of two teenaged girls, my once-proud Johnson the size of a peanut, gritting my teeth so as not to start crying and screaming.

At least they didn't giggle.

After the catheter was out, which took about ten seconds but felt like about four months, they brought a little white plastic tub and told me to pee in it as soon as I could. Thankfully, I accomplished that only a few minutes later and the urine was blood-free. Dr. Porter told me he would push the pathology through as quickly as possible, and that I would probably have the results the following Tuesday. I cleaned up, got dressed, and Laura guided me unsteadily to the car.

Chapter Five

The weekend passed quickly. I spent lots more time reading about bladder cancer, but I also went cycling with my friend Jeff, went to Sunday morning spinning class, and spent time with the family. I was concerned about the results, but surprisingly calm and unstressed, given the stakes. Tom Petty's "The Waiting Is the Hardest Part" was my mental musical background. As it turned out, I didn't have long to wait. Dr. Porter called me on Monday afternoon. He was far too serious and professional to use the old "I have good news and I have bad news" opening, but that was the gist of it. First off, he told me I definitely, 100% certainly, had bladder cancer. Then came the big surprise. He had removed the tumor all the way, as deep as it had penetrated, and he was surprised to see that even though it was large and definitely Grade III, it was still contained in the mucous membrane and had not invaded the muscle wall. So the tumor was officially T1 Grade III, and my official diagnosis was high-grade T1 urothelial (transitional cell) carcinoma. So, on Monday, November 5th, 2007, I became a cancer patient.

Chapter Six

Over the next several days I once again immersed myself in information. I came to the slow realization that there were and are two distinct and opposed schools of thought regarding treatment for organ-confined bladder cancer. The first, the bladder-sparing school, is also known as the East Coast or Sloan Kettering school, named after the famous New York cancer hospital where the TURBT procedure was perfected. They believe in radical surgery only for the most advanced cancers, as a last resort after all other options have been exhausted. The second school of thought is the radical surgery school, also known as the West Coast or USC Norris school. They believe that the only reasonable course of action in most T1 or higher cancers is removal of the entire bladder. I'll get into the details presently.

Of course, one of the first things I asked for when we got the results of the TURBT was a second opinion. Dr. Porter sent me to see a well-known Seattle urologist at Virginia Mason Medical Center, coincidentally also named Porter, Dr. Christopher Porter. He was actually my third opinion, as I had accompanied my wife to her regular checkup with her oncologist, Dr. Kathryn Crossland, at Overlake Hospital in Bellevue, Washington. Both Drs. Porter II and Crossland strongly recommended that I not rush into any further surgeries, agreeing with Dr. James Porter that I should heal up for five or six weeks then undergo a second TURBT to make sure there were no hidden tumors. This would be a much better evaluation, since the original tumor and all the associated blood would be gone. It was clear to me that all three doctors were firmly in the bladder-sparing school, which was not surprising to me.

But Dr. Christopher Porter took it further. He rather forcefully told me to beware the radical surgery proponents. He called them "evangelists" for their particular surgery, and even implied that they wanted to cut every patient that they saw. His advice was that I not let any of them near me with a knife! You might expect that this would have pushed me even further into the bladder-sparing camp, but the opposite happened. What was so different about their radical surgery approach that would inspire such passion in the opposing school? I resolved to find out.

A week after the TURBT, I returned to Dr. James Porter's clinic for a follow-up. All was well, and at the end I told him I wanted to seek a fourth opinion, and that I wanted it to be someone who was committed to the radical surgery approach to bladder cancer treatment. He told me that there really weren't any true bladder cancer specialists from that side in Washington State, and cautioned that my insurance would probably not cover out-of-state appointments or procedures. I said that was the least of my concerns and that I would go anywhere for the right doctor. He then told me that probably the best bladder cancer surgeon in the world was at Oregon Health and Science University (OHSU) just three hours south of Seattle in Portland, Oregon. He told me he knew this doctor personally; in fact, they had been on opposite sides of the bladder cancer debate at several medical conferences.

"I'll answer the question you haven't asked," Dr. Porter said. "If there was something wrong with my bladder, this is the man I would call." I asked him if I should call him, and he said he would do that for me, as this doctor was backed up for months and only took a certain kind of patient. Dr. Porter said he thought there was a reasonable chance that my case would be of interest to him.

The surgeon's name at OHSU was Dr. Sia Daneshmand.

DECISION

Chapter Seven

D r. Porter obviously followed through on his promise to contact Dr. Daneshmand at OHSU, as his office called me around 10:00 a.m. the next day. His receptionist told me he was interested in my case, and in fact had already requested that the original pathology slides of the removed tumor be sent to him. She explained that he only worked from the actual slides, not any other doctors' third-party reports. She told me the slides were being couriered down to Portland that very day. She asked me how soon I could be available to come down to OHSU. When I answered, "Three hours," she laughed and said, "Well, how about Thursday around noon?"

And so on Thursday morning I found myself driving down I-5 to Portland alone. My mind was all over the place, and I suddenly remembered an episode from about six weeks earlier that I had completely forgotten. I don't particularly believe in the occult or paranormal experiences, but I do believe that sometimes we just "know" things. I had inexplicably awakened at about 3:15 a.m. and was lying on my back with my hands clasped behind my head staring into the darkness when Laura woke up and asked me if something was wrong. I answered her with words that surprised me as much as they did her, because I had not even thought them before they emerged from my mouth.

"There is something inside of me," I said.

"You mean something in your mind?"

"No. Something is in my body. Something is wrong, and I have no idea what it is."

We went back to sleep with no further discussion, and I promptly forgot about it until that moment in the car. It was obvious to me now that somehow I had sensed the cancer inside me, even though I had no physical discomfort or pain of any kind prior to the blood episode. A chill went through me as I tried to imagine what my next course of treatment would entail.

Chapter Eight

I arrived at the OHSU Center of Health and Healing, which is where the doctors have their offices and clinics, at about 11:15 a.m. on November 13th. The sixteen-story building sits at the base of a hill on the South Waterfront in Portland. A modern cable car runs from the Center to the top of the high hill at the summit of which is perched the vast OHSU hospital and university. The urology clinic was on the tenth floor of the Center, and I checked in and waited, tense to say the least. I had been told to expect several hours of tests and interviews, and not knowing what procedures were likely and what kind of shape I would be in afterwards, I had reserved a room at a downtown Portland hotel.

My appointment started out innocuously enough, with a friendly female nurse checking height, weight, blood pressure, and temperature. After that, I was introduced to Mark

Johnson, Dr. Daneshmand's primary nurse. I didn't realize it at the time, of course, but this was another of those pivotal moments, as he and I hit it off immediately. He was very professional, but had an easygoing disposition and a caring bedside manner. He took me through extensive questioning, on medications, general health, and medical history, as well as what seemed like psychological profiling. I was very comfortable talking with Mark, and I became increasingly relaxed and confident.

The next phase was a complete physical. I met one of Dr. Daneshmand's assistant surgeons, Dr. Eric Reid. He was an energetic young man with a broad smile, and I liked him immediately. He had read all of my questionnaires and immediately focused on my listing cycling as a main hobby. He asked about my work with the Lance Armstrong Foundation (soon to be re-christened Livestrong) and we chatted about Lance for a bit. I told him he looked a little bit like Lance, and over the ensuing months I would come to call him Lance. He explained that we were going to do a "full" physical that would take some time. I'll spare you the details, but suffice it to say that Dr. Reid and I became much closer than two heterosexual males should ever be.

Following the physical I enjoyed a short break. It was nearly four in the afternoon, and I had eaten nothing since breakfast at home in Sammamish. I went down to the café and got a yogurt and a big bottle of water and returned to the waiting room on the tenth floor. A short time later I was called back and placed in a small examination room to wait for the doctor. I was tired but very pleased with everyone I had encountered throughout the day and quite confident in their abilities. I waited there for about a half hour, and then I met the amazing Dr. Daneshmand.

Dr. Sia Daneshmand had earned his medical degree at the University of California, Davis, and completed his residency at the University of Southern California (USC), followed by a two-year fellowship in urologic oncology at the USC Norris Comprehensive Cancer Center. He had been at OHSU for just over four years, and had established the Section of Urologic Oncology as a center of excellence for the treatment of bladder and testis cancer.

He strode into the room with a big smile. A diminutive guy, dressed in a sport coat over a tieless dress shirt and slacks, he shook my hand vigorously, thanked me for coming down, and apologized for the long day. He asked how the nurses and Dr. Reid had treated me, and I told him I was most impressed. Then we got down to business. He confirmed the diagnosis of a T1 Grade III malignant bladder tumor, using the pathology slides he had received from Swedish in Seattle the day before. We then embarked on a long discussion mainly centered around statistics. We talked about recurrence rates, survival chances, and the typical progress of this type of disease. I told him about the consistent advice I had already received from no fewer than three doctors, who all advised a bladder-sparing strategy involving a second TURBT and a biotherapy treatment called BCG. This treatment involves filling the bladder with weakened tuberculosis bacteria once a week for a six-week period, and has been shown to decrease the recurrence rate in early-stage bladder cancer. He listened to all this carefully, and pushed back with what would become the defining statistic in my treatment decision. Between 25% and 35% of all T1 tumors are in fact misdiagnosed muscle-invasive T2 disease. The therapy for T2 bladder cancer is immediate removal of the bladder, since the disease can break out of the bladder and become fatal T3 cancer literally at any time.

We talked in more detail about recurrence. I learned that bladder cancer has the highest recurrence rate of any cancer, in the range of 50-80%. It requires life-long surveillance, which is why it is the most expensive cancer to treat on a per-patient basis. It is not hyperbole to say that you will know you are cured of bladder cancer when you die from something else.

We spent about ninety minutes reviewing all of this, and I told him that from everything I had seen and heard I was sure I wanted him to be my doctor going forward, regardless of what treatment we would decide upon. After more conversation he asked me point blank how I wanted to proceed. I told him that I thought the most prudent course would be to follow Dr. Porter's advice, taking a few weeks to recover before having a second, investigative TURBT. At that point we would have a better idea of whether there was more cancer involved. Dr. Daneshmand's response stunned me. He told me that he respected my decision no matter what it was because I was dealing from a position of knowledge, but that he could not be my doctor. He explained that he had more patients than he could possibly treat, and that even though my case looked like just the type he favored, he could only treat those who he judged to be 100% committed to doing everything possible to achieve the highest likelihood of survival. I told him that's exactly what I thought I was doing, and that's when he laid it out in plain English.

"This thing is only in your body for one reason," he said. "It's there to kill you. You can play offense and you still may die. But you might not. If you play defense like the other doctors are recommending, you will almost certainly have continued recurrences until one becomes metastasized and kills you."

He went on to describe each part of the treatment regimen that the bladder-sparing guys were recommending, presenting the statistics for each. He pointed out again the almost inevitable recurrence, the one-third misdiagnosis rate for T1 tumors, and the 50% maximum effectiveness for BCG therapy, not to mention its frequent side effects. I realized he was making a lot of sense.

I swallowed hard. "So what should I do?" I asked, half knowing the answer.

"You should get on my surgery schedule just as soon as possible and have your bladder removed."

I was speechless for a long moment. I said that I supposed his recommendation was based on the frequent misdiagnosis of T1 cancers, but what if I had my bladder removed and it turned out that I was one of the two-thirds who did not have hidden T2 disease? He said without hesitation that that would be the best possible outcome. Needless to say, I had a hard time wrapping my brain around that one.

"But it would mean that I really didn't need to have my bladder taken out!" I protested.

"Look at it this way," he said. "If it was truly only T1 disease, you have an almost 80% chance of recurrence. Plus, at one-third misdiagnosis you are literally playing Russian roulette … with a three-shooter."

Recovering a bit, I then asked him about the surgery. I said I assumed that I would have a hole in my side and an external bag for urine. He said that was certainly an option and a possibility, but that there were other options, such as a neobladder. I had never heard of this, and he began to explain it to me in some fairly technical medical terms. It was at this moment that a nurse came in and told him he was needed in another exam room for a few moments. He excused himself, and I sat by myself in shock and terror. Even though I had known he was from the surgery side, I didn't think this was how this day was going to go. Dr. Reid knocked and entered. He told me he understood that Dr. Daneshmand was beginning to explain the neobladder option. I said that was true but I really didn't understand it yet. He sat across from me on the stool where Dr. Daneshmand had been sitting and put his chin in his hands, elbows on his knees.

"Here's what we do," he said. "We cut you from stem to stern, and take out your bladder, prostate, seminal vesicles, and thirty to fifty abdominal lymph nodes. Then we cut out a one-meter section of your small intestine, the ileum, still alive and hooked up to the blood supply. Then we use the intestine to build a new bladder in the cavity where your original bladder came out. We hook one end up to your kidneys, the other end to your exit pipe, and you're good to go."

I was completely floored that an actual doctor had put it in such terms. Dr. Reid looked at me and winked.

"Actually, Frank, it's just a little more complicated than that."

Chapter Nine

When Dr. Daneshmand returned a few minutes later, he resumed his explanation of the surgery he was proposing. It was pretty much exactly as Dr. Reid had paraphrased it; a new bladder would be constructed from my own body tissue. I told him that I would need to talk to my wife and think about it for twenty-four hours or so. He said of course, and the day was over. It was after six o'clock. I had been there for almost seven hours. I was yawning as I retrieved my car from the underground garage and drove to my hotel. When I got there I called home and gave Laura the long version of the day. She was encouraged that I thought so highly of Dr. Daneshmand and his team, but expressed her concern that he was asking me to jump into exactly what I had been so emphatically warned against: a quick decision to undergo radical surgery.

We had lived in Portland from 1999–2001 before moving

to the Seattle area, and I had lived in a company apartment downtown for five months before the family moved out there, so I knew downtown Portland very well. It was a typical November night, forty degrees or so with a light, steady rain. I walked up to Broadway and then north a half-dozen blocks to Higgins, one of the best known Pacific Northwest "farm to table" restaurants. I can't remember eating, but I guess I did, and an hour or so later I was back on the wet streets, walking down Salmon Street to the Willamette River waterfront. I walked the length of the Tom McCall Waterfront Park on the west side of the river and crossed the Steel Bridge to the East Side Esplanade. It was getting late, but there were plenty of Portlanders out on a rainy weekday night—walkers, runners, and bikers, all oblivious to the steady rain. I walked on, pondering my situation. Was I ready to put my faith and possibly my life in the hands of a doctor I had met less than ten hours earlier? It was hard to grasp, but the more I turned his statistics and his logic over in my head, the more sense it made.

I returned to the hotel sometime after 2:00 a.m., took a hot shower, and fell asleep quickly, to my surprise. I woke without an alarm at 6:15 the next morning, and felt amazingly well rested. A weird feeling of calm and confidence had come over me. I was also starving. As I ate bacon and eggs and drank good strong Portland coffee, I realized from where my calm confidence was coming. I had made my decision without consciously knowing it.

I would put my life in Dr. Daneshmand's hands, play offense, and have the surgery.

Chapter Ten

My call home went as well as could be expected. Laura pledged her support of whatever course I chose, but I could detect the uncertainty in her voice. I told her that she needed to meet Dr. Daneshmand and his team to really understand why I was so confident in the decision.

My next call was to Dr. Daneshmand's office. I spoke with his receptionist and told her I had made a decision concerning my treatment. She cut me off and said Dr. Daneshmand would definitely want to talk to me in person. I gave her my Blackberry number, checked out of the hotel, and began the three-hour drive back to Seattle. I was about an hour up the I-5, just past Longview, Washington, when my phone rang. I pulled off onto the shoulder and hit my flashers before answering. This was a call that merited my full attention. I told Dr. Daneshmand that I wanted to move

35

forward with the radical surgery option, and asked him if he had a time frame in mind. He must have been pretty confident of which way I would go, as he said he had already looked at his surgery schedule. He gave me two choices. The earliest he could squeeze me in was less than four weeks hence, on Friday, December 21st. He pointed out that this schedule would have me in intensive care on my birthday, December 22nd, and in the hospital for Christmas. The alternative date was Friday, January 4th. During our conversation the previous day, he had repeatedly stressed the urgency of starting whatever course of treatment I decided upon, due to the Grade III, fast-growing tumor that had been removed. I brought this up and asked why I wouldn't pick the earlier date. He mentioned sensitivity to the holiday season, and I laughed out loud. "I'm not at all concerned about *this* Christmas," I said. "It's the next ten I'm worried about!" He laughed too, and it was set.

THE BIG CUT

Chapter Eleven

The next three weeks were a blur. The first Monday I returned to New Jersey and informed my company of the situation, explaining the seriousness of the diagnosis and the nature of the surgery. They agreed to give me a ninety-day leave of absence and then to play it by ear going forward from there. On Wednesday I quickly packed up my apartment, putting most of my belongings, including my East Coast guitar and bike, into my SUV. I boxed up the kitchen, bathroom, and bedroom items, and took the whole lot over to a garage-sized storage unit that I had rented the day before. Two of my direct reports helped me with the move. I canceled all of my upcoming international travel, and spent half a day sending quick, ambiguous emails to the company folks and vendors with whom I would have been meeting over the following ninety days. Thursday night I said some emotional goodbyes to my boss (the CEO of the company), my direct reports, and lastly, my loyal executive assistant, Michele.

That Friday I flew back to Seattle, where I would remain for three and a half months. I was greeted by a thick envelope with the return address of OHSU in Portland. It contained a bewildering array of documents, beginning with every manner of release followed by extensive patients' rights, responsibilities, and safety documentation. Next was a twelve-page, single-spaced document titled:

Radical Cystectomy
(Removal of Urinary Bladder)
Cystectomy with ileal conduit
Or
Cystectomy with neobladder

It was authored by Sia Daneshmand, MD, and Mark Johnson, RN, of the Bladder Cancer Program at Oregon Health and Science University. Mark would become very important to my bladder cancer journey, as you will read in the pages and chapters ahead. With paragraph headings like "Continent Orthotopic Diversion," "Radical Cystectomy with Pelvic Lymph Node Dissection," and "Catheter Care and Irrigation," this document became my most important resource for really specific information in the days before the surgery. I had one additional long conference call with both Dr. Daneshmand and Mark Johnson, and we went over it paragraph by paragraph, with both of them providing additional details based on their extensive experience as well as pointing out where some of the most difficult recovery points were. A three-page appendix called "Neobladder Irrigation" detailed the required care and feeding of the new bladder, and the four-page follow-on called "Instructions and Follow-Up" was a detailed summary of what to expect in the estimated three weeks of preliminary recovery at home with catheter and surgical drains. To be honest, the whole thing was beyond daunting; for the first time since I read the survival statistics, I was truly freaked out. The thoroughness of the clinical detail made me realize that I was heading for an extremely complex procedure that inevitably would produce major physical, mental, and emotional trauma in my person. I was nervous and I was scared, but I can honestly say that I never once second-guessed my decision to go with Dr. Daneshmand's radical surgery program. Of course it had been a difficult decision, but once I was in, I was all in.

Chapter Twelve

On the night of December 19th, two days before the scheduled surgery, I began the "bowel prep" process designed to completely clean out my digestive system. From that point on I was to have only clear liquids the entire next day, and nothing at all the morning of the surgery. As a guy who is well known as one who loves his food, this was more difficult that I would have thought. I was starving! After driving down to Portland that afternoon, we had an early "lunch" at Sinju Japanese restaurant in the Pearl District, where we now live years later. While Laura somewhat guiltily noshed on maguro and hamachi nigiri, I slurped down two bowls of miso soup, being careful to filter out the small cubes of tofu and just take the broth.

Our daughter-in-law's mother and stepfather live in Vancouver, Washington, just across the Columbia River from Portland. They graciously offered to put up the family, which consisted of Laura and the younger two of our three children, in their house through my hospitalization. As for Laura and me, we had decided to spend the night before surgery in a downtown Portland hotel, both to be close to OHSU early the next morning and also to spare everyone night two of my bowel-prep regimen.

You're welcome.

The next morning we rose early and headed for OHSU hospital, at the top of the big hill known affectionately by Portlanders as "Pill Hill." We didn't say much. I have no recollection of the weather on the morning of December 21st, 2007. I was feeling exhausted and a bit woozy, literally and figuratively drained by the long preparation. We arrived at the hospital and got checked in easily and quickly. Everyone was super-nice, but it was obvious by the quiet voices and short conversations that they knew this one was a big deal. It was at this point that an almost preternatural calm came over me. As they started an IV and made me comfortable in the pre-op area, I was not the slightest bit nervous or concerned. I was so relaxed that when they told me they were going to inject a mild sedative into my IV so I would not be anxious, I joked that I might pass out and miss the whole show. I did mention that I was incredibly thirsty, and told them I was concerned about dehydration. They assured me that they were hydrating me with the saline IV and that I would be able to have ice when I made it to recovery. Here's where I would ordinarily crack the obvious joke, "You mean, *if* I make it to recovery." But not today. Today I was calm, relaxed, and trusting that the best bladder cancer surgeon in the world was on his way to the operating room with me.

After twenty or thirty minutes, Mark Johnson came in and asked me how I was doing. I told him everything was fine and that I was ready to get my disease behind me. He put his big hand on my shoulder.

"That's the way to look at it," he said.

Chapter Thirteen

Just a few minutes later, Mark came for me. I said good-bye to Laura with a smile and a kiss, and they put me on a gurney and wheeled me through a short maze of hallways to the operating room. Just as I was going down the final stretch to the doors of the operating room, I had a totally bizarre thought. How were they going to get to my bladder? Were they going in from the front of me or through my back? This must have been drug-induced, because I had not only seen umpteen detailed drawings of the surgical process, but Dr. Daneshmand himself had also traced the likely line of the incision on my bare belly in demonstration. To this day that remains one of my most inexplicable and bizarre thoughts.

I remember, vividly, entering the operating theater, a line of white-scrubbed nurses and physicians, gloved and ready, standing to my left. It was freezing cold, and they covered me with two soft warmed blankets. Dr. Daneshmand entered. I could tell by his eyes that he was smiling even though his mask covered his mouth.

"Mark tells me that you're doing very well with all this," he said.

I answered in the affirmative, and he told he had one more introduction to make, to the anesthesiologist. Actually to the team of anesthesiologists, as this was to be a protracted surgery. He asked me if I had any questions. I had been reading everything I could about the surgery, and I understood that the anesthesia for long surgeries was different from that for routine operations. As I had been reading so much about bladder cancer and surgeries in general, I had been exposed to a phenomenon called "anesthesia awareness" that is reported widely on the Internet. It involves miscalculation of anesthesia dosing where the patient actually wakes up and feels the pain of the surgery. During long surgeries, patients are given a combination of a paralytic and a memory eraser, and there are many documented accounts of patients awakening during surgery but being completely paralyzed and thus unable to signal their distress. So I asked the anesthesiologist whether I would be asleep throughout the long surgery. He told me that technically I would not be asleep, but he immediately knew where I was going with the question. He asked if I was talking about the "urban legends" of people feeling pain, or the actual documented dosing errors. I said both, and he assured me that not a single one of his or any of OHSU's anesthesiologists' patients had ever awakened during surgery, and he promised me with "100% certainty" that I would not be the first. Thus reassured, I relaxed and took a last look around the operating room, calmly taking in the machines and tools that were laid out in front of the surgical team. Dr. Daneshmand put a hand on my shoulder.

"Are you ready, Frank?" he asked.

"Yes."

He nodded at the anesthesiologist, who said, "Here we go."

And there I went.

Chapter Fourteen

As reported in the Prologue, it was around 4:00 p.m. when I finally came to, in intensive care. My surgery had taken almost eight hours, and Dr. Daneshmand pronounced it a total success. He had built me a new bladder out of my own body parts. The full medical name for the procedure I had undergone was "radical cysto-prostatectomy with orthotopic ileal neobladder and extensive pelvic lymph node dissection." Quite a mouthful! As mentioned earlier, the decision on which urinary diversion would be created was not made until the surgery was well underway. As they prepared to remove my bladder, they first disconnected it from the ureters coming down from the kidneys and the urethra on the other side. They then snipped a small section of the ureters and urethra and rushed them to the pathology lab as a biopsy. It was only after the biopsies were determined to be completely cancer-free that the decision was made to proceed with the neobladder.

I was in and out of consciousness for that first evening, and in some significant pain that was mitigated by large IV doses of Dilaudid. They had put a port in my neck, which gave them instant access to a vein for infusing whatever they needed to give me without multiple IV's, for which I was very thankful. I became very aware of the large diameter catheter that was draining urine, blood, and copious amounts of mucous from the new neobladder. I also had a surgical drain coming out of my right side that was draining the area around the incision, but that was not painful, just a little uncomfortable. Later that evening I was even clear-headed enough to talk to my parents in Florida for a few minutes. Thinking back on it, I must have sounded like a total druggie, as I was going on and on about how great I felt—and I was, in a word, euphoric. It was the Dilaudid, for certain, along with the increasing awareness that I had in fact made it through the surgery. I figured that the worst of my cancer experience was now solidly behind me.

Little did I know.

Later that first night, just before my exhausted wife left me to get some much-deserved rest, the nurse came in with a strange-looking device. A brief digression: In the late 1980's, Sony introduced a line of electronics products designed and built for children called "My First Sony." Products included an amplified microphone, boom box, cassette player, clock radio, and headset walkie-talkies, all in bright colors and having big, easy-to-use buttons. The color scheme was a distinctive red and yellow. So when the nurse came in with this device, the first thing I noticed was that the cylinder with a button on top was in the exact color scheme of My First Sony. When I learned that there was in fact a large button that would trigger a self-administered dose of Dilaudid to be released into my neck port, I laughed uncontrollably. Further proof that I was doped to the gills. I looked at the bemused nurse, who had asked me exactly what was so funny.

"It's 'My First Heroin,' " I said in between guffaws, thinking it was the single funniest thing anyone had ever said.

But then I got the bad news: it was only good for one dose every fifteen minutes. I will confess to watching the clock tick off the last four or five of those fifteen minutes many times throughout that first night. I also had developed temporary diabetes, which apparently is fairly common after long surgeries, so I was awakened every hour to have my finger pricked to check my blood sugar. For these reasons I did not really sleep much, and I greeted the next day, December 22nd, my fifty-fifth birthday, in a fog of drugs and exhaustion. My wife was there early to check on me, and my spirits rose upon seeing her. I told her, not entirely truthfully, that the pain had been under control through the night. I was ready for day one of my recovery.

It was at about this time that I realized that I had virtually no feeling in my thighs, except for a pins-and-needles feeling on the front of both legs. This worried me, especially when they came to get me up walking, which I knew was essential to recovery. I was concerned that I would collapse when I tried to stand on legs I could not feel. They wanted to take me for an MRI immediately, which I refused, wanting to talk to Dr. Daneshmand. He arrived very shortly thereafter and told me what I was experiencing was a bit unusual but not unheard of. We agreed to wait until his late afternoon rounds to decide what to do next. As it turned out, when the physical therapist came around in the early afternoon to see if I was able to get up, I had a bit of feeling coming back and was able to take a few steps into the hallway outside my room in ICU, with the nurse pushing the IV tree that was feeding me some cocktail of saline and antibiotics through my neck port. She had Velcro'd my urine bag to my right calf and pinned the surgical drain's reservoir to my so-called gown. I'm sure I was quite a sight shuffling out the door with my tubes and bags.

I had been briefed in detail on what to expect over the first few days, so it was no surprise that they wanted me up and walking right away. I knew that this would help speed up the process they called "waking up the bowels," which is just what it sounds like. To say the removal of a meter of small intestine to create the neobladder had confused my digestive system would be a colossal understatement. The plan was to keep me on clear broths and thin soft cereals until I had some type of movement in the digestion. You get the idea. At that point it would be safe to move to some more nutritious food.

I continued to take short walks every few hours, and I headed into night number two in ICU with a good deal of optimism. The pain was manageable, and the every-four-hour irrigation of the neobladder was not at all painful and considerably less awful than it sounds. They started me on breathing exercises with a clear plastic device called a spirometer that offered resistance to my inhalation and exhalation, which would gradually strengthen my lung function, which was explained to me as being critically important to recovery. I went at it with a vengeance, surprising the nurses. I have no doubt that my cardiopulmonary fitness from years of cycling was the reason for my impressive lung power. At this point I was extremely tired and was looking forward to a better night's sleep.

That was not to be. First there was the blood-sugar tests' every-hour finger stick. After a lifetime of sleeping on my stomach, sleeping on my back with the catheter draining at my side was pretty uncomfortable too. Then at what I would guess was about 2:00 a.m. there arose a ferocious amount of urgent calls and running footsteps, all centered on the room next to mine. This lasted for over a half hour and pretty much wrecked my sleep plans. I learned the next morning that the patient in the next room had died during the night. For privacy reasons, no one would answer my questions about what had happened to him or her— whether it was post-surgery, a traumatic accident like a car crash, or something else. In any case, it brought the reality of intensive care home for me, and I realized how fortunate I was to be recovering normally. I spoke to my parents, and even had a visitor, my good friend Roland and his fiancé, who came into the ICU briefly. Unfortunately, I picked that time to suffer one of the bouts of intense nausea that came with the return of digestive function. I politely asked them to leave just before I threw up violently and repeatedly.

Chapter Fifteen

After two days and nights in ICU, the team was pleased enough with my progress, particularly the walking, that they were ready to have me transferred to a regular room. I was moved without incident and placed in a large double room in another wing of the hospital. The second bed was empty. Two of our three children were staying with Laura at the house in Vancouver, and they came to visit me in my new room, which cheered me immensely. I noticed right away that the hospital bed in the new room was nowhere near as comfortable as that in the ICU, but due to the Dilaudid, and my exhaustion from the surgery and lack of sleep in ICU, I did manage to get some rest that night. The next day was Christmas Eve.

I awoke early the next morning and for the first time felt hungry. I realized that other than the broth and the two cups of miso soup I had had days back, I had really eaten

nothing for the better part of a week. I also felt the first stir-
rings in my gut. The bowels were awakening! As it turned
out, nothing would actually happen on that front until the
next morning, but Dr. Daneshmand was encouraged and
said I was right on schedule. I had a great Christmas Eve
visit from the family, and although I was increasingly uncomfortable in the new bed, I felt like I was making real
progress. I was being weaned off the strong painkiller, with
both the dose and the frequency becoming less and less. I
was not in any serious pain at this point, and my spirits
were high. Little did I know that going into Christmas Day I
would experience the first of many low points in the recovery process.

After the family left sometime in the late evening, I settled in for what I hoped would be a restful night. My
stomach and lower intestines continued to roil and rumble,
which I knew was a positive sign, but sometime after mid-
night I was wide awake, feeling hot and clammy at the same
time. I realized that I just could not get comfortable in the
bed, and that I was suddenly ravenously hungry. I pushed
the button and summoned the nurse on call.

Another brief digression. I have already been pretty clear
about my feelings about Dr. Daneshmand and his team,
particularly Dr. Reid and Mark Johnson. I can now say that
virtually everyone I met on the OHSU staff during my initial visit, my hospitalization, and my follow-up care was
absolutely fantastic—friendly and professional to a "T."
There was one exception that proved the rule, the nurse on
duty overnight on Christmas Eve. It was painfully obvious
from the first time I summoned her that she absolutely did

not want to be there. I certainly can't blame her for that, but her bedside manner was awful. When I told her the bed was so uncomfortable that not only could I not sleep but I literally wanted to scream, she curtly informed me that all the beds in the ward were absolutely identical so they weren't going to do anything about it. When I complained of hunger she gave me a downright condescending sneer, pointing to my chart.

"It says right here that you are allowed clear broths at mealtimes. This is not a mealtime. My job is to follow this chart and I am going to do just that," she said, turning on her heel and striding out the door. After another ninety minutes of writhing around on the bed, literally in tears, I pushed the call button again. This time she entered visibly angry, and essentially told me to suck it up and stop being a baby. After all, who doesn't expect discomfort after major surgery? I could not believe her mean attitude, and I did not summon her again.

I find it quite interesting that none of what she told me was actually true, as I soon found out. After a truly horrible night, I was as close to despair as I had been since learning the survival rate for T3 bladder cancer weeks before. Shortly after 6:00 a.m. on Christmas Day, the day shift nurse came in and cheerfully asked me how I was doing. She was the same nurse from the day before. As she spoke, she took a real look at me and stopped short.

"What is the matter?" she said, hurrying over to the bed. She had been really helpful the previous day, and had such a concerned tone now, that I just let it all spill out. I told her of the supreme discomfort I experienced all night in the new bed, how I was ravenously hungry all of a sudden, and that I felt I was near emotional collapse. Tears were rolling down my cheeks. Finally, I told her about the attitude of the night nurse. She was astonished at the way I had been treated and apologized on behalf of OHSU. Then she lifted the corner of the mattress and looked closely at the bed.

"Oh my God," she said, "this is one of the really old beds that have all been replaced. Obviously they missed this one. I'll have them bring up a brand new bed right away and change it out. And with regard to the food, it is true that you are on primarily clear liquids, but there is no rule that you can only eat at meal times. In fact, we are specifically told to bring approved nutrition at any time of the day or night when the patient requests it. In your case, having an appetite is a great sign of recovery, and your body is crying out for nutrition."

She immediately brought me a big bowl of steaming chicken broth and a cup of decaf green tea. I think it was the most delicious meal of my life. Soon after that, the new bed arrived.

Less than a half hour later Dr. Daneshmand came in on his morning rounds. He was not pleased, to say the least, as the day nurse had briefed him on my rough night. He apologized again for the poor treatment and asked me about my digestion. I told him about the rumbling and movement, and he asked me if I had passed any gas. I said I had, and he suggested I head to the bathroom and make an attempt. There was a small success, and he told me that I would have crackers with my broth, a bit of cream of wheat cereal, and best of all, scrambled eggs the following morning.

Merry Christmas!

Chapter Sixteen

With my good spirits restored, I accomplished my longest walk to date—three laps of the ward—and had a wonderful extended Christmas visit from the family. I ate three packs of crackers with my beef broth, and immediately had another restroom success. The new bed was really comfortable, totally different from the antique that I had, and I anticipated a good night's sleep with a full belly and a working digestive system. I was grateful for the turnaround, but keenly aware of the very short distance between being thankfully comfortable and in the depths of despair when recovering from traumatic surgery.

Christmas night came without incident after my evening laps around the ward, and I slept soundly for the first time since the surgery. I was awakened very late by the sounds of the nurses moving a patient into the other bed in my room. They were behind a curtain dividing the room and were trying to be quiet, but I was again wide awake. The new patient spoke in a shaky voice and seemed old, or weak, or both. He had a raspy voice and a smoker's cough. I could feel his terror. I heard them tell him that they would be checking on him hourly and that Dr. Daneshmand would see him first thing in the morning. I was hoping for his sake that it was not bladder cancer, but if it was, at least he had lucked into the best in the business.

At about 6:30 a.m. I heard Dr. Daneshmand's voice from the other side of the curtain, speaking in a low but serious tone. It was a speech I had heard before. He was talking about the grades and types of bladder tumors, their likely causes, and the treatment options. His family joined the party a short time later. The patient seemed very confused and kept asking how they knew he had cancer. His daughter told Dr. Daneshmand that her father was a lifetime smoker and had lung problems. I never did find out what kind of episode landed him in the hospital, but he was discharged late that day, presumably with an appointment to have a TURBT. I flashed back to my own TURBT with Mr. Serious, Dr. Porter. Was it possible that that it was less than eight weeks ago?

I continued to walk several times a day, the family visited, and I ate very small quantities of bland food. Surprisingly, my appetite had deserted me, even though I was feeling better. The day after Christmas I was completely off the Dilaudid, and that afternoon they removed the port from my neck. That meant an IV, but at that point I had been sliced, poked, and prodded so many times that I really didn't notice it much. Also, the surgical drain was not particularly uncomfortable and not painful at all. What I did notice was the catheter, which was becoming increasingly uncomfortable as the days passed. I knew from my pre-surgery briefings that I would have it in for approximately three weeks after my release from OHSU, and I wondered how it would be toting that thing around the house, and of course trying to sleep. Laura would be in charge of the every-four-hour neobladder irrigation process, and I was concerned for her as it promised to be stressful caregiving.

Later that day Dr. Daneshmand came around for his late rounds and announced that I would be released the following morning. So on Thursday, December 27th, six days out from surgery, they packed up all my medical gear and irrigated the neobladder one last time. I said goodbye to the nurses and Dr. Daneshmand, and they wheeled me out to Laura's waiting car. I remember turning to Laura and saying something to the effect of, "Getting home to our own bed will be heaven."

Wrong again.

HELL

Chapter Seventeen

I was both uncomfortable and exhausted on the three-and-a-half-hour ride back to Sammamish from Portland. I suppose I dozed off a few times, but I was acutely aware of the catheter and the urine bag Velcro'd to my calf. I also had periods of intense nausea, but thankfully I never made use of the bucket on the floor of the passenger seat. When we got to our home, Laura and our son Craig helped me to carefully exit the car in our garage. It took some time, but I was able to successfully navigate our back stairs, with a lot of help. I headed straight for bed, but immediate sleep was not an option. Four hours had passed from the irrigation the nurse had performed before checking me out, so we had to have our first try at it right away. It involved disconnecting the catheter from the urine bag, loading up an injector that looked exactly like a turkey baster with sterile saline solution, and injecting the saline into the neobladder. This would dilute the mucous created by the piece of ilium used for the bladder. Then the injector would be removed and the saline and mucous would drain into a handy bucket. It had not been painful when they did this in the hospital, but they were professionals. Plus I had never actually watched in the hospital, so I was pretty apprehensive. Just like most of the procedures I had been through, the whole thing sounds considerably worse than it actually was. I will allow that it felt pretty weird, but it was not painful in any way, and Laura did it flawlessly on her first try. I will spare you a literary description of what wound up in the bucket.

A pretty decent nap followed. I was very concerned about accidentally pulling on the catheter, but I had been sleeping with it for the better part of a week in the hospital, so I lay on my back with it snaking down to the bag on the floor to my left and I passed out. I was taking oxycodone and Advil every three hours, so I was not in a lot of pain.

It was night when I awoke, and Laura brought me some food, which I could not bring myself to eat. I have never been a soda drinker, but I had a strong craving for a Coke. Mark had mentioned that non-diet sodas would be a decent source of some sugar calories if I had difficulty eating. Over the next weeks I would consume more Coca-Cola that I had in my entire life to that point.

The nausea came during that first night home. I threw up so fast and hard that I did not even have time to lean over the bucket. I heaved so violently that I thought I would rip the incision open. I was dizzy and more nauseous than I had ever been, and thus began a pattern that was to last for the better part of two weeks: violent vomiting that came on with absolutely no warning, followed a half-hour or so later by equally violent diarrhea that arrived the same way. What a mess! I remained dizzy and somewhat disoriented for the next forty-eight hours, waking up with Laura every four hours for the irrigation process. I slept fitfully, unused to sleeping on my back, which was necessary with the catheter and drain. I was completely exhausted, more tired than I had ever been or could have possibly imagined. I thought I must surely have hit the bottom.

Wrong, yet again.

But the bottom was not far away. After two days I was starting to realize when the diarrhea was coming on, if not the vomiting, which was still pretty spontaneous. It was this that had me in the bathroom late in the afternoon on Saturday, December 29th. While doing my laps around the upstairs rooms, I would carry the urine bag in the big side pocket of my heavy terrycloth bathrobe. When I was in bed, sitting in a chair, or on the toilet I would lay the bag on the floor at my feet to help the neobladdder drain more easily. But this time I made a very bad mistake. I did not realize that after I laid the bag on the bathroom floor I had moved my feet while sitting down so my right sandal was on the catheter. When I was finished and stood up, I wound up giving a very hard yank on the catheter because I was standing on it.

A searing pain like nothing I had ever felt tore through me. I screamed and fell forward flat on my face. Tears poured down my cheeks and I thought I would pass out. Laura heard the scream and was instantly at my side asking what had happened. I croaked out an explanation as best I could, wondering exactly what kind of damage I had done to the drainage system. I also noticed that the almost continuous drip of salmon-colored urine through the catheter had stopped, and I thought the worst. What I didn't know was that the pain and anxiety were sending me into shock, causing my blood pressure to literally collapse.

Chapter Eighteen

My account of the next few hours and days is my best memory of the events, aided by the detailed records that Laura was keeping and the reports from various doctors. I am sure my memories differ significantly from those of folks who were in much better shape than I was. For example, I have a very distinct memory of regaining consciousness at some point after the accident lying on the carpeted back staircase to our second floor, feet facing down. Laura, who was at my side constantly, disputes that I was ever even on the back stairs after the accident. Apparently I gently tried to push the catheter back in, but it was too painful. Then I tried to "walk it off." Yeah, right. The result of that desperate move was that I passed out and fell in the hallway. At this point I was pretty much delirious and constituted two hundred pounds of totally dead weight. My athlete son was not at home to help Laura get me up, but she and I somehow managed to move me about fifteen feet into our oldest son's unused bedroom. I don't remember much of this, but Laura's records say that she called a Dr. Wagner at 5:40 p.m., about a half hour after the catheter incident. Paramedics were called, and arrived shortly thereafter.

When the two guys—I'll call them Laurel and Hardy—arrived, they asked me a few questions. From my frayed answers, they quickly concluded that I was in poor shape. A check of my blood pressure showed it to be dangerously low, and the rest of my vital signs were going haywire. They not-so-gently rolled me onto a stretcher, strapped me down, and carried me down the steep stairs with difficulty. Our next-door neighbors, who had seen the lights of the ambulance, were looking on in horror in our entry hall. I gave them a thumbs-up as I passed, but I'm sure I looked like death itself.

The paramedics put me in the back of the ambulance, and as we pulled out they started to discuss what they should do about my condition. It was not confidence inspiring. Laurel talked about various drugs they might give me, and Hardy was concerned with what they would do if I went into cardiac arrest from the blood pressure issue. I pointed out to them that I was in fact right there and could hear everything. One thing that the comedy team agreed upon was to start an IV and keep me hydrated. Now remember, I had just endured an eight-hour surgery, drains, catheters, a port implanted in my neck, hourly finger sticks, and more IV's than I could easily count. But the needle they brought out to start this IV was the biggest I had ever seen.

Because of my dehydration, their incompetence, or most likely both, neither Stan nor Ollie could find a vein. And the monster needle hurt like hell. It was on the fourth or fifth try that it blessedly slipped into a vein. They patched the other bleeding holes and told me we would be at Swedish hospital in about fifteen minutes, the same hospital in which I had spent the night after my first incident with the blood, and where I had initially met the good Dr. Porter, a.k.a. Mr. Serious. My addled brain tried to cope with the events since that visit that seemed so long ago, but I was not processing data very well, so I just let go and passed out.

Chapter Nineteen

I awoke as Stan and Ollie were carrying me out of the ambulance and into the emergency ward. Laura had followed and was once again back at my side. They wheeled me into a treatment room and we waited for the doctor on duty. I regained enough coherence to remind Laura of Dr. Daneshmand's admonitions about the catheter. It was a special catheter, he told us, which had been inserted deep into the neobladder and secured with an inflatable balloon at its end. A regular emergency room doctor would assume it was a standard "Foley" catheter that could just be pulled out and reinserted. He had told us that if anything happened to the catheter the doctor treating me was to call him directly at any time, day or night.

After a few minutes we met Dr. Eric Hartman. Laura quickly explained that I had been through surgery and had a neobladder with a complicated catheter. He examined it closely. There was still nothing coming down the pipe, and I was getting increasingly concerned. I couldn't imagine what would happen if they couldn't fix this. Would the backed-up urine damage the neobladder? Would it burst and kill me? Would I be medivaced to OHSU for more surgery? The room was spinning when Dr. Hartman decided to try to gently push on the catheter, which elicited a scream of agony from yours truly. Even the attending nurse was near tears, and said, "Doctor, you have to give this man something for the pain before you move that catheter."

"Yes, of course," he said. "Give him a unit of Dilaudid in the IV."

She prepared it without delay and injected it into my IV line. The effect was almost instantaneous but I was still in considerable pain, sweating profusely. Laura begged him to call Dr. Daneshmand and he left the room to do so. When he returned he was grim-faced but determined. "I spoke to Dr. Daneshmand at length," he said, "and he has given me detailed instructions on how to deflate the balloon and re-position the catheter." I was waiting for the doctor-speak about "mild discomfort" but to his credit he didn't bother. "This will be painful," he said. "Nurse, give him another unit of Dilaudid." He also told me that due to the low blood pressure and dehydration he had strongly recommended that I be admitted to the hospital immediately. Dr. Daneshmand had just told him, however, that that would be the worst possible thing for my recovery, and that I needed to be at home. He also predicted that my vitals, including blood pressure, would return to near normal as soon as I knew the catheter was back in place and I was rehydrated.

The Dilaudid hit me hard, and Dr. Hartman deflated the balloon without incident. But when he started to push the catheter back into place, the pain became unbearable, and he reluctantly gave me another unit of Dilaudid before continuing, informing me that there was no more where that came from. I was at the maximum safe dose, even for a big guy like me. In minutes the procedure was over, and the sight of bloody urine flowing down the pipe was one of the most beautiful things I had ever seen. I lay there for another ninety minutes as they let two half-liter bags of saline drip in. As predicted by Dr. Daneshmand, my blood pressure stabilized only slightly lower than normal, way out of the danger zone. The doctor wrote me prescriptions for strong antibiotics, fearing infection, and started me on them before releasing me. A wheelchair brought me to Laura's minivan, and once again I headed home, with bag and drain as my companions.

Chapter Twenty

The night of my return from the catheter accident trip to Swedish hospital was the start of the strangest and most surreal forty-eight hours of my life. I was blasted to the moon on Dilaudid, pumped full of high-powered antibiotics, and as deeply fatigued as I had ever been in all my fifty-five years. I went straight to bed. My account of what happened to me that night and the next day comes from my best recollections, but I am sure much of it is pure hallucination. At the time it was all too real, and it terrified me.

Maybe I slept. Maybe I didn't. Thoughts began to swim through my brain with strange patterns. I would seemingly fall into a deep sleep only to dream dreams I will never remember, then gradually awaken through a series of hypnotic, psychedelic visions with impossible sights and sounds. At about 4:00 a.m. in the pitch dark, the visions resolved into a series of what I can only describe as TV screens. There were always more than one, and always "playing" something different. It started as contrasting patterns of colors on two, and then a row of three, of these screens. Over the next half hour, more screens appeared, eventually resolving into nine separate "programs" in three rows of three. They remained whether my eyes were open or closed in the darkness.

The images began to change, morphing one screen at a time from moving patterns of colors into images and snippets of what looked like TV shows. Some were clear and in focus, some were behind a curtain of old-time TV static, and still others were out of focus and out of proportion like a funhouse mirror. I saw people that I knew and strangers, places that were vaguely familiar and strange alien landscapes. I had no control over these moving images, and I began to be very afraid. I tried hard to reassure myself that they were caused by the drugs and fatigue, and that as soon as it started to become light I would regain control. This gave me little solace, and I spent the next two hours literally shaking with fear.

As the first light of pre-dawn came through my bedroom window, I summoned what little strength I had and tried to mentally shut down the images, eyes wide open and staring at the brightening window across from my bed. A new chill of fear shuddered through me. Even in the light, I was powerless to stop the visions.

I was losing my mind.

The visions continued on and off throughout the day as my sense of dread increased. Would I be like this for the rest of my life? I guess somewhere deep inside my brain I must have known it was a temporary condition, but the feeling of helplessness only added to the fear. One of the most frightening aspects of this period is that I was apparently mostly coherent to those around me, except for some periods of disorientation. I remember talking to Laura while she diligently irrigated the neobladder every few hours. I remember her telling me we were discontinuing one oral antibiotic that I had been taking post-surgery and starting a stronger one. At some point, I believe in the morning, Dr. Hartman called from Swedish hospital. When Laura described my condition, he implored us to come back so that I could be readmitted to the hospital for observation. But the argument was the same one we had been through the night before, with Dr. Daneshmand's recommendation trumping Dr. Hartman's. He begged us to reconsider. I remembered the commitment I had made to Dr. Daneshmand and his methods when I made the decision on the neobladder surgery.

"Thank you for your concern, I really appreciate it," I told Dr. Hartman. "But I'm all-in with Dr. Daneshmand, and I'm sticking with his plan." Dr. Hartman told me one last time that I was making a big mistake and signed off. I have the greatest respect for him, because I know his actions were out of a genuine concern for my well being. I have never had occasion to speak with him again.

Chapter Twenty-One

As the second night approached, I was in and out of the hallucinatory visions that I call the "screens." I was terrified of completely losing control again during the night. I was to learn that we all have mechanisms inside of our minds that engage in the worst of times. For some it's a rediscovery of lost religion. Others focus on their family ties as their touchstone. Still others just get mad and use their anger to overcome their helplessness.

For me, it was music.

From the time I was in grade school, I was always in a band. I started out as a drummer until halfway through high school, when a strange situation made me discover my true musical love, the guitar. My roommate and fellow band member, guitarist Mike Pecht, had fallen hard for blues harmonica after I discovered a book called *Blues Harp* by Tony "Little Sun" Glover. Since Mike played guitar, I had a ready-made accompanist as I tried to learn harmonica. He soon tired of this as I progressed faster than him, and he demanded that I learn at least a three-chord blues in the key of E on the acoustic guitar so I could accompany his harmonica efforts. I did, and I've been a guitarist ever since.

In 1971, while in college, I formed a band with my roommate, who was just starting to learn the drums, and an accomplished blues bassist who lived in the next dorm over. We eventually added a talented lead singer and began to play frat parties and other small gigs. Over the next several years, we added and subtracted members but kept that core group, and we graduated to nightclubs and the outdoor festival parties common at the time. We played both covers of famous bands' songs and lots of originals, most written by me. To combat our utter lack of discipline, we took to a system of grouping songs that we used to make practices more efficient and later extended logically to our live shows. We would group three or four songs together that totaled as close to fifteen minutes as possible, then played them in that exact order, with no breaks between the songs, every time we practiced. They were little mini-sets that we called "presets." We would call them by the name of the first song in the preset. Since virtually all of the gigs we played were some number of forty-five-minute sets, making the night's set list was as easy as selecting three presets per set. We used this system for years.

As I lay in bed in my darkening bedroom, the hallucinations returned with a vengeance and my pulse rose quickly. The screens were multiplying and going crazy with colors, distorted live action, and noisy static. The fear that I was actually, literally, losing my mind returned in spades.

And then, from somewhere, I thought of playing live with the old band. I latched my mind onto the thought like a drowning man grabbing a lifeline. I focused on the top left screen with all my might, and almost cried when I saw the first four frets of my first electric guitar, a 1969 Fender Stratocaster, appear. Suddenly, I knew the first preset we played nearly every night needed to start. Three songs from the Velvet Underground: "Waiting for the Man," "White Light, White Heat," and "Sweet Jane." The other screens winked off one by one, and I focused on the one remaining, seeing my fingers land behind the frets, making the basic E-major chord that begins the first song. I heard the intro clearly as I dropped my pinky on the third fret of the B string to make the chord E7, and I heard the throbbing bass line take us up to the A chord and back to the E. Exhilaration flowed through me as I looked to my left as I had done so many times, hearing the first lines of the strong vocal.

> "I'm...waiting for my man
> Twenty-six dollars in my hand.
> Up to Lexington, one-two-five
> Feel sick and dirty, more dead than alive."

The irony of these lyrics about a drug buy was completely lost on me. I only know that I simultaneously felt a huge rush of strength as well as the lifting of a great weight from me. I blew a chord on the chorus and forgot the words to the second verse, but I was laughing inside anyway as I started again. I have no idea how many restarts I needed or how long it took until I made it to the crashing final chords, but when the last chord was silenced I heard the three sharp drumstick clicks of the drummer counting off the next song, and we were flying into "White Light, White Heat."

Throughout the night, I pushed through the first three songs over and over until I got all three right, forcing my fingers to accurately make the chords and play the fills and leads that we had practiced for so long. I pushed into preset number two—three Rolling Stones songs—and sometime the next day, after getting those right, came the first three original songs. An idea was forming in my head, and I was getting excited.

By the third day after my emergency visit to Swedish hospital, I had settled on a mock "Greatest Hits" concert of two forty-five to fifty-minute sets plus an encore. We had often talked about a reunion concert over the years, but it had never happened. Suddenly, here it was. I felt like I had been practicing ten hours a day even though I had not put finger to fretboard other than in my mind. I continued to polish the sets, making a few minor song changes and adding two completely new cover songs; I also somehow wrote a short acoustic song to serve as a final encore, kind of a coda to the concert. This all may sound pretty weird, but I fully believe that the focus on that old music brought me back from the precipice of mental breakdown. It was serious stuff to me, and it also served to steel my resolve to recover completely from the surgery. I now had purpose. And the screens were gone.

Chapter Twenty-Two

The next two weeks were fairly brutal by any standards. Although I had conquered the hallucinations and terrors, I had virtually no ability to keep any food down. Everything tasted terrible, and I lived on Coca-Cola and potato chips. I would eventually lose over thirty pounds in just under a month. I was still throwing up, if only occasionally, but my bowels were becoming a bit more predictable. I was able to speak with my parents on the phone a few times, but the fatigue was indescribable. As a lifelong pro football fan, I would shuffle into the upstairs media room on Sundays and try to watch a game, often accompanied by my youngest son. Invariably, I would find myself staring at the wall behind the big TV, unable to follow the game or even recall who was playing.

I had few visitors during this time. Only one of our three children was still living at home, and he was busy with high school and basketball. One of my great regrets is that he had to see me during this period of my recovery, walking endless laps around the upstairs in my thick white terry robe, surgical drain pinned to the front and a long tube snaking to the urine bag in my pocket, growing more gaunt by the day. There was one person who visited me regularly, and this book would not be complete without a bit about him. His name is Jeff Smith.

I met Jeff in the late 1980s when we both worked at an electronics and appliance retailer called Silo in Philadelphia in the merchandising division. I was the head of the audio buying team and Jeff managed computer products. Eventually we would work together at four different companies across the country, finally ending up together in Seattle working for Amazon, where I was the head of consumer electronics merchandising and Jeff was in charge of digital cameras and camcorders. Throughout the years we were always cordial, sharing the occasional cookout with our families, but we were never really close friends. What bound us together was our mutual love of cycling. We spent a lot of time together on the road, riding for hours through the cornfields of Ohio, climbing the West Hills of Portland, and plying the foothills of the Cascades out of Sammamish. We have ridden over 10,000 miles together. Even after Jeff trained for a Tour de France cycling tour and became a hugely strong rider, he always had the time to "grab a loop" with me on one of our many routes around Sammamish.

When I was diagnosed with advanced bladder cancer, Jeff was dumbstruck. I joked that he was more upset by the whole thing than I was. As soon as I returned home following the big surgery, I started receiving hilariously irreverent get-well cards every two or three days from Jeff. He became my only regular visitor outside of the family. When I was at my worst, he would stop by and sit at my side, either in the bedroom when I was too weak or on the big couch in the media room if I was walking. We would share stories of some of our "epic" rides as well as the latest news from the professional cycling circuit. He brought snacks and food, but quickly realized that I wasn't eating, so he seamlessly switched gears. It became a running joke that exists to this day. He brought me water.

First there was Perrier and San Pellegrino and Fiji. Then it got increasingly exotic. He would show up with Calistoga or Voss, Gerolsteiner or Volvic, then odd little six-packs of small blue bottles, the names of which I cannot remember. Since both of us were also avid wine drinkers, we would have a few potato chips and taste the latest water, expounding on the nuances of flavor and texture as though it were a fine Bordeaux or Burgundy. To say that Jeff's visits during this period helped keep my spirits up would be a huge understatement. If you ever want to find out who really cares about you, just get cancer.

Chapter Twenty-Three

In those first few weeks at home, Jeff had been my only real visitor. He would come over and sit with me so my long-suffering wife could have a bit of time away from the monotony of the caregiving. Sometime during week two at home, I had the best surprise of all. I had just completed a seemingly endless series of laps around the upstairs, and I was resting on the couch in the media room with my ubiquitous bowl of chips and a bottle of very fancy water. The door to the hallway opened, and my oldest son Keith walked in. It was a total surprise. He had taken a couple days off from his job at Cirque du Soleil and flown up to Portland from his Las Vegas home. I was happier than I had been in a very long time. Tears flowed down my cheeks as we hugged. It was then that I realized how much my family's support meant to me during this most difficult recovery. Seeing my son was the single most uplifting event of the entire cancer experience. After his visit I attained a totally different level of resolve, committing myself to work even harder. I was going to get well.

Keith's visit did something else, too. I realized that neither of my two sisters had come to visit. They never did. When my wife had cancer a few years earlier, almost everyone in her family made the cross-country trek to support her. Since we've become adults, my sisters and I have not been particularly close, and my parents were too old and frail to make the long trip, but I still get a strange empty feeling when I think back on that period with no family visitors other than the children. The phenomenon of long-time friends and even family vanishing from cancer survivors' lives is an unfortunately common one. I will deal with it in more detail in a later chapter.

Chapter Twenty-Four

The days slowly passed. I still had very little appetite and was plagued by digestive turmoil and the overwhelming fatigue. I did start to crave some other foods, and my dinner became an iceberg lettuce salad with a simple vinegar and oil dressing around the beginning of my third week at home. I was still eating chips and drinking Coke the rest of the time. I was showering regularly and feeling a bit more human. Needless to say, I was exceedingly careful with the catheter, especially in the bathroom and in the shower. I still had tape covering the incision, which ran from just below my sternum, around my belly button, to just above my pubic bone. I would later affectionately call it my "Guinness Book of World Records scar." The cards and visits from my friend Jeff continued, and one day short of three weeks after leaving the hospital in Portland, it was time to go back for the next steps.

FOLLOW UP

Chapter Twenty-Five

Early on the morning of January 15th, 2008, I got dressed in sweat pants and a loose-fitting shirt, pinned the drain to the shirt, and carried my urine bag out to the garage, where Laura's minivan waited. We had a noon appointment at OHSU in Portland, which would consist of a general check-up, blood and urine tests, and a cystogram to look at the neobladder. If all went well, the catheter and drain would then be removed. Finally, we would have a discussion with Dr. Daneshmand and Mark Johnson about how to proceed with the next stage of recovery.

The drive down was far less uncomfortable than the ride home three weeks prior, but I was tired and very, very sick of the catheter and surgical drain. We arrived at the clinic building of OHSU, the Center for Health and Healing, a little over three hours later. Since we were almost an hour early, we got some tea from the coffee shop downstairs and went up to the urology waiting room on the tenth floor of the modern building. Mark came out soon after we checked in and asked how I was doing. I told him I was tired but anxious to finally have the pipes taken out of me. He directed us to the correct floor to get started with the blood work and urine sample. I remember thinking how anxious a simple blood draw made me just a few months before. Now, after having just about every possible thing stuck into me, I was completely calm about these first tests. Not so the cystogram.

A smiling Dr. Daneshmand greeted us in the waiting room just before 1:00 p.m. and led us back into the treatment room. After a short conversation about my progress and a quick look at my incision, which was healing nicely, he prepared me for the cystogram.

There are basically two types of tests that give a doctor a look at the bladder, or in my case the neobladder. They are both invasive. The first is called a cystoscopy, and involves the insertion of a large-diameter catheter into the urethra and up into the bladder. There is a fiber optic camera and light at the end of the instrument, enabling the urologist to visually scan the interior of the bladder close up. The second test involves a regular catheter, which is used to inject a contrast solution into the bladder. Then an external scanning device projects images of the bladder onto a large high-definition video screen in real time. The doctor manipulates the angles and views and creates digital captures of the images he wants to keep.

In my case, I should have thought about it a bit more. If I had, I wouldn't have been so nervous, since I already had the catheter in place! All they needed to do was drain the neobladder thoroughly and introduce the contrast fluid through the existing catheter. It was exactly what we had been doing every few hours at home for the past three weeks. It was not at all painful, just a bit uncomfortable as they filled the bladder to capacity to get accurate images. I confess it was a bit strange to be looking at the new bladder in real time and in color, but Dr. Daneshmand was very obviously pleased with what he saw.

"It's perfect," he said, pointing out the size and shape of the neobladder and the attachment points of the ureters and the urethra. "Just about perfect for three weeks out."

With everything looking good on the cystogram and the blood and urine tests coming back negative for cancer as expected, it was time for the main event. The removal of the catheter and the surgical drain. I was taken to another examining room and laid on a gurney. Mark Johnson was to do the procedures. He started with the drain, warning me that it would hurt but only last a few seconds. He popped the stitches that had held it in place since the surgery almost four weeks earlier and after a countdown warning he pulled it out in one smooth motion. It was a sharp pain, but not close to the worst I'd been through, and it lasted only a few seconds. Honestly, it felt great to have it out of me.

Then it was time to lose the catheter. Mark deflated the balloon and began to try to slide the catheter out. He had told me that it might be uncomfortable but that I should feel no sharp pain. When he began to move the tube, I involuntarily cried out in pain so severe that sweat burst out on my beet-red face. He tried one more time with the same result: excruciating pain. He stopped and looked down at me.

"This is not going as planned. I am going to get the boss."

Dr. Daneshmand walked in a few minutes later, absent his usual cheery smile. He had obviously conferred with Mark. He took hold of the catheter just a few inches from its exit point and pushed it in and out maybe a half inch. He saw and heard the result—more sweat and another scream. At this point there were six people in the room, not including me: three young female students, about whom I had long since ceased caring, my wife Laura, and Mark and Dr. Daneshmand. The good doctor looked around and said quietly, "I'd like everyone to leave the room for just a few minutes."

"Even me?" Laura said.

"Yes, it would be best."

I knew at that point that it was probably not going to be a whole lot of fun in that room. Dr. Daneshmand pulled up a stool and sat down, looking down at me on the gurney with concern in his eyes.

"Here's how it is," he began. "What has happened is that the balloon end of the catheter has become folded back on itself, which is causing the pain when we attempt to slide it out. It's like it's obstructing itself."

"So what do we do?" I asked in a shaky voice.

"We have two options," he said. "We can put you on the tram up to the hospital, admit you for the night to give us time to line up an anesthesiologist, and put you under tomorrow morning and take it out. You wouldn't feel a thing. But of course you wouldn't be going home this evening like you had planned."

"And the other option?" I was not sure I wanted to hear the other option.

"The second option is that I just go ahead and pull it out," he said. There was no nonsense about "mild discomfort" at this point; he told me it would hurt like hell.

"But it'll be quick, it won't injure you, and you'll be fine to go home in an hour or two."

"Define 'quick,'" I said.

"Ten seconds, tops," he said, "and probably more like half that, say, five or six seconds."

At this point, the absolute last thing I wanted was to be admitted to the hospital, so I figured I had no choice if I wanted to get home.

"Do it," I said, sounding a lot braver than I felt.

"OK," he said, "but you cannot make any kind of jerky movement when it's happening. That will make it much worse because I'll have to stop and start again. You can scream, though. That will help."

So, with another countdown, he removed the catheter in one continuous motion. I screamed bloody murder for the longest six seconds of my life, but then it was out and there was just a lingering ache that a few Advil would take care of. There was some blood and mucous, but he seemed satisfied that he had not mortally wounded me. He sat back down on the stool, and I thought I detected moisture in his eyes. He put his hand on my shoulder.

"I am so very sorry that I hurt you like that," he said.

Was this guy the best, or what?

Chapter Twenty-Six

I had been told before the surgery what to expect when the pipes came out. First, incontinence. Every neobladder patient goes home from this follow-up in a diaper. It's like starting life over as an infant as far as your urinary system is concerned. So I was prepared for that. What I was not prepared for was what I was required to do before I could be released.

The neobladder is a piece of the ilium, or small intestine, that has been reshaped into the new bladder. As intestine, it produces mucous, and for the first months it produces *lots* of mucous. This mucous has been known to clog up the pipes sufficiently to require irrigation. The docs don't want you running to the emergency room every few days, so before they release you, you are required to demonstrate that you are able to catheterize yourself and flush the neobladder with sterile saline.

Yes, you read that right. *Catheterize yourself.*

"Surely you jest," I said to Mark when he informed me an hour after the pipes came out that this was next. Actually, what I really said was more like, "Mark, you have got to be shitting me, dude! I just had a folded up garden hose yanked through my crank an hour ago, and not to put too fine a point on it, but it *hurt*!"

"You have to do it to get released," he said. "You do want go home, right?" Oh, I get it. Hardball time. "And it's really not as bad as it sounds."

"No?" I said. "So let's see you do it first."

Needless to say, that was not going to happen, so I figured it couldn't possibly be any worse than the catheter removal I'd just been through and I'd better do it. So Mark gave me the instructions on how to prep the catheter, and myself; handed me one in a sterile paper wrap; and passed me a tube of KY-like catheter lube. It burned like hell going in, but I learned one thing right away. Catheterizing is way easier when you no longer have a prostate, which tends to be the big barrier and causes 90% of the discomfort. Having been catheterized multiple times prior to my surgery, I noticed the difference right away. Once it was in place, it was a simple and painless thing to fill the device that looked like a big turkey baster, attach it to the funnel end of the catheter, and flush it out. There was a lot of mucous and a little leftover blood from earlier, but it was surprisingly easy and straightforward. I tried to copy the smooth, seamless withdrawal I had learned earlier in the day with both the drain and catheter. Oh yeah, and it burned like hell coming out, too.

Chapter Twenty-Seven

The second-worst day of my life was almost over. After cleaning up and donning another huge hospital diaper, I got dressed and waited in yet another examining room with my wife. Mark came in and said there was only one thing left; Dr. Daneshmand wanted a short conversation before they released me. I was filled with dread when I saw his unsmiling face come through the door. He sat on a stool across from me and told me there was one more serious discussion needed. At this point I was badly hurt and unbelievably tired, and I immediately assumed the worst: he was here to tell me I still had cancer.

"We need to talk about the pathology," he began. When they remove the bladder and the other organs, they are extensively tested for additional signs of cancer. I immediately assumed that they must have found cancer cells in one or more of the thirty-eight abdominal lymph nodes they had removed, which would indicate that the cancer had escaped the bladder after all.

"First of all, " he continued, "I want you to know that we found absolutely no evidence of any cancer outside your bladder. Every single lymph node was clean." My relief knew no bounds, and I felt as though I was about to lose it and just break down and cry.

"But ...," he said, and it sounded like the biggest and worst "but" ever. "We did find a second tumor in your bladder. It was a T2 Grade III tumor, muscle invasive, but organ confined. It was hidden behind the cauterized layer of tissue from your TURBT, and was millimeters from the external bladder wall. If you had gone the bladder-sparing route, or actually if you had even delayed the surgery, it is highly likely that you would have had T3 disease." I knew all too well what that meant, and now I did fall apart and cry.

After a few minutes I composed myself somewhat and looked tearily across at his face. His smile was back.

"You saved my life," I said.

"You made the hardest decision of your life, and no doubt the best. So, no, Frank. I did your surgery. You saved your life."

RECOVERY

Chapter Twenty-Eight

The long ride back to Sammamish was tiring for sure, and I was very uncomfortable in the bulky diaper, but it was a happy ride. My emotions were all over the map, but the main ones were a huge sense of gratitude for the expertise and wonderful caregiving of the team at OHSU, and an almost physical sense of joy at having another chance at life. I knew it was going to be a long hard road back, but I was upbeat and dying to get started on a real recovery. Laura asked why I kept smiling.

"It happens automatically every time it dawns on me again that I don't have those pipes in me any more."

We made a quick pit stop at the drug store near our home to pick up some of the maximum-capacity Depends undergarments. According to Mark, I would need them for a week or two before I could switch to the thinner and much more comfortable standard Depends. In a completely unspoken agreement, we have never again referred to them as diapers. They will be forever known as "adult absorbency products." I am very grateful that humor has been a big part of this journey from day one.

It was great to get home, and especially as I was now un-encumbered by the drain and catheter. I had been carefully counseled by Mark to be patient with all aspects of the recovery, but most especially the two that every radical cystectomy patient is most worried about: incontinence and impotence. I knew that everybody went home in a diaper, and that progress was different for every patient. In the first years of neobladder surgery, a period of six months to up to two years of daytime incontinence was normal, and nighttime continence was frequently double that or longer. In many cases nighttime continence was never achieved at all.

Additionally, just to make things interesting, there is the phenomenon known as hyper-continence. This condition, while far less common, does happen to some percentage of patients, and particularly to women. It is the inability to pass urine at all, and requires regular self-catheterization on a schedule. Although it is usually a temporary condition, there exist a significant number of cases where catheterization is the permanent necessity.

So one of the keys was to be patient and not give in to the natural frustration that an adult feels when he or she has no bladder control. Incontinence can wear you down emotionally, eat away your self-esteem, and even lead to serious clinical depression, none of which is conducive to recovery. So I followed the advice of the team, timing my efforts at regular urination at about every two hours. This was necessary because I could not tell when I had to go. The normal bladder is a muscle, and the stretching of that muscle is the feeing of "fullness" and urgency to urinate. This does not exist with a neobladder, as it is a piece of intestine. Eventually, most neobladder owners, myself included, recognize and develop an entirely different sensation that enables them to know when they need to go. If I could describe it, I would, but it's just a totally unique sensation that only neobladder patients understand. Over the years, Dr. Daneshmand and a few other top bladder cancer surgeons had increasing success, so much so that his average neobladder patient achieved full daytime continence in just a few weeks. Nighttime was always going to be more difficult, but the results there were also impressive.

Over the next few days, I tried mightily to not let my incontinence get to me, but to be honest I was only partially successful. I had made a major personal commitment to my recovery, and I was very anxious to see some concrete results. Over the first four days, I saw little improvement, and frequent accidents.

As part of the recovery regimen, I was told to irrigate the neobladder with sterile saline every other day for the first two weeks. This involved self-catheterization, draining of any urine, and the injection of saline through the catheter with the turkey-baster device. The purpose was to flush out any thick mucous clumps that could clog the urethra and cause a trip to the emergency room. To say I dreaded this process would be the understatement of the century. I couldn't stop thinking about it all night before the alternate days, and I worked myself up into a fairly high state of anxiety beforehand. I must admit that the thought of it was much worse than the act itself, which I was able to perform without issue in just a few minutes in the morning before my shower. The catheter was not painful, and neither was the irrigation. It was doubtless just the unnatural nature of the act itself that bothered me so.

After the third catheterization and flushing, on the sixth day, I realized that barely any mucous was coming out with the saline. In fact, I had far more mucous come out—easily and painlessly—during regular urination. I phoned Dr. Daneshmand's office after completing the irrigation, and he called me back personally a couple of hours later.

I told him what was happening, and he said, "That's great news. You can stop catheterizing completely unless you notice you're not passing mucous when you urinate."

I assured him I would be paying close attention, but that I was passing significant mucous every single time. Another large understatement would be to say I was happy with his advice.

Chapter Twenty-Nine

During this period I took great joy in being able to walk outside. Even though it was winter in the Seattle suburbs, I got out at least once or twice a day in addition to walking indoors, even going up and down the stairs. The first day after arriving home I dressed warmly, very carefully negotiated the front steps and sloped driveway, and did the little-old-man shuffle down to the corner—about forty yards—and back. On day two I went about twice as far, and day three saw me make my first walk around the block, about a third of a mile, even including a small hill!

By day four I was walking a mile outside, and had transitioned from the bulky maximum-capacity adult absorbency products to the regular slim Depends. For the first time, it felt a whole lot like progress.

I didn't know it at the time, but there were to be no other

major setbacks. By day five after my return home I was urinating vigorously every three hours. I still couldn't tell when I needed to go, but there were no accidents and leakage was infrequent. As it turned out, I was daytime incontinent for only five days. From day six until today I have been 100% daytime continent, which is a very short time, even by Dr. Daneshmand's high standards. This destroyed once and for all any chance of my becoming frustrated over any other aspect of my recovery. I was quite simply ecstatic at the hard evidence of improvement. Even though I knew I had a long way to go, my optimism and enthusiasm knew no bounds after just one week at home and unfettered.

Chapter Thirty

[The next short section of this book is about sex. If this subject gives you a case of the yips, you may want to skip the next few pages. I don't think it appropriate in this type of book to go into the clinical details, so I won't. If you are a bladder cancer patient or caregiver and wish to discuss the actual, intimate details, feel free to contact me directly and I will be happy to share. My contact info is in the "Acknowledgements" section at the end of this book.]

The second thing that concerns every guy who has ever undergone a radical cystectomy is impotence. Of course, it varies from guys who absolutely obsess over it to guys—usually older—who simply don't care. The average age of bladder cancer diagnosis in men is seventy-five, so there are more of the latter than you might think. I was diagnosed at age fifty-four, so you can probably guess where I fell on the spectrum: realistic but concerned. Fortunately, Dr. Daneshmand and his team are as progressive in this area as they are in the continence arena, which is to say as progressive as anyone in the world.

In the early days of neobladder surgery, lifetime impotence was simply the price paid for not having the stoma and external bag. When Dr. Daneshmand's mentor started to perfect the operation, he instructed his surgeons to learn the nerve-sparing surgical skills of the top prostate surgeons and to apply them to the prostate-removal portion of the neobladder surgery. This nerve-sparing is absolutely essential to the rehabilitation of sexual function.

During the meetings prior to the surgery, Dr. Daneshmand, Mark Johnson, and Laura and I had some very frank discussions about sex. They explained all of the options for regaining potency. There are pills, suppositories, pumps, shots, and implants, usually tried in roughly that order. At fifty-four and very happily married, sex was important to us. Of course, although quality of life was important to me, my number one concern was always saving my life.

So we put together a fairly detailed plan. Like the incontinence issue, it was very important to not get frustrated and depressed. With the delicate nature of the male ego in the ED arena, this is even more important than in the area of incontinence. The operative concept here was "use it or lose it." You couldn't just wait for the capabilities to return on their own; you had to work at it. Even if it was frustrating and unsuccessful, you had to keep trying. Being blessed with an incredibly patient and loving wife made all the difference in the world for me, and although I can't say I am 100% the "old me" even today, we were able to resume a real sex life less than eight weeks after my return home.

Chapter Thirty-One

Now I got better fast. Within two weeks, I was walking two miles twice a day, and my appetite was returning. I was able to add a bit of lean chicken breast to the ubiquitous iceberg salads and even had a scrambled egg some mornings. However, my digestive system was still a wreck, having a mind of its own. It didn't seem to matter what I ate. I would just spontaneously lapse into an inability to keep anything in me, what we would come to refer to as my "digestive meltdowns." Also, even though I was clearly gaining strength, the fatigue was still very debilitating. On the plus side, I was able to sleep much better without the tubes, although I did need to get up every three hours to urinate. Even with that schedule, I was barely continent for more than a night or two in a row. I was not too discouraged about this, thanks to the excellent pre-surgery counseling from Mark Johnson and my quick success with full daytime continence.

At 10:00 in the morning about ten days after my return home, our doorbell rang. I opened the door to find a delivery truck parked out front and a deliveryman with a clipboard standing next to a huge wooden crate. It was for me. I signed for it and Laura and I carried it into our entrance hall. I laid it down and saw that the top was carefully secured with screws and marked as the "open here" point.

Retrieving the electric screwdriver, we carefully opened the crate. Inside, nestled in a molded Styrofoam enclosure, was a large, airline-ready guitar case. I gently lifted it out, and there was an envelope affixed to the top of the case. I opened it. The card inside said, "From your friends at D&M Holdings. If you play this every day, you will get well soon."

The guitar inside was a small-body acoustic that is often called a "parlor" guitar. On the headstock, the brand was simply "Goodall." I was blown away. James Goodall is one of the most famous luthiers (stringed instrument makers) in the world. He is based in Maui, Hawaii, and custom makes each instrument to order. I knew where this one came from. My boss, the company CEO and a friend for over twenty-five years, had several Goodalls on the wall of his music room. It was a gesture of consummate generosity, as this instrument ran over eight thousand dollars. He called me a couple of days later and asked me how I liked it.

"I have a house full of guitars," I said, "but I only have one work of art." I played it every day for months, and I've been playing it regularly ever since.

As the days became weeks, I continued to feel more like a human being. Although I was down thirty pounds from my pre-surgery weight, my weight had stabilized and I was no longer dropping a pound or more a day. I was starting to taste food again, and I began to slowly broaden my diet. I was even venturing a glass of mild white wine with my chicken dinners, and eating some cooked veggies as well.

Chapter Thirty-Two

February 9th, 2008, is a day that will live in my memory forever. It was a cold, sunny Saturday morning in Sammamish, and I was feeling great. My strength was returning in dramatic fashion, and the fatigue at long last was becoming manageable. I had gone for a brisk walk all the way to the entrance of our development and back, about two miles, and I was having a cup of green tea in the family room upstairs. I was on my way down the hall to visit the bathroom when I looked down at the driveway from the hall window and saw my friend Jeff's Honda minivan in the driveway.

"Is Jeff here?" I called downstairs to Laura.

"Yes, he is," she said in a voice that sounded, well, pissed off.

I quickly went down the stairs. Looking into the garage, I saw Jeff, in full winter cycling gear. His Litespeed Classic titanium road bike was propped against the wall, and he was energetically pumping up the tires on my Trek Madone carbon fiber ride.

"Better dress warm," he said. "It's sunny, but it's cold out there."

"No."

Laura walked up behind me.

"No," she said.

"Oh, but yes," said Jeff. "It's time."

"If he crashes and messes up the surgery, Jeff, I will literally kill you." Guess who.

"He'll be fine," Jeff said. "We're just going for an easy spin around a few blocks."

And so I went. I walked my bike gingerly down the sloped driveway to our street, which was a very gentle downhill left to right. I pushed off, coasting down the road, and carefully clicked my cycling shoes into the "clipless" pedals. It felt so amazing to be riding again that tears filled my eyes. Of course, I claimed it was from the cold breeze. About two hundred yards down, we made a left turn and went up a very small hill, about 150 yards at only a 3% or 4% gradient. When we were out riding together months before, we'd stand up and ride over it while chatting, not even bothering to shift gears. By the time I reached the top this day, I was in my lowest possible gear and sucking wind like I had just climbed a two-mile, 10% hill. Our joke about that first ride has remained the same.

"Other than the eight-year-old girls with training wheel bikes passing him on the hill, Frank did pretty well."

We went three miles that day, at an average speed of

about 10 mph. I felt pretty great about the whole thing, but I couldn't help but think back to the 2005 Ride for the Roses in Austin, Texas. That's the Lance Armstrong Foundation's signature annual event, and we attended for many years. In 2005 I had logged over 3,500 road miles on the bike and was in the best cycling shape of my life when the October date rolled around. I weighed 184 pounds at the start, and completed the hilly 108-mile course at a personal best 20 mph average speed. Would I ever be able to ride like that again? In a hot shower after Jeff had gone home, I vowed to myself to ride the Ride for the Roses in October 2008. I had no idea what I was getting myself into.

During the protracted rainy season, I returned to my spinning classes. Over the next weeks, even though I was getting stronger on the bike, I realized that I would likely never be the rider I was before cancer. It made me very sad. By May, as the rides got longer and the weather better, we attempted some of the climbs that I breezed over in years past. I had never suffered like that on the bike, ever. Where we used to bang out fifty to sixty-five miles on a weekend ride, I felt myself hitting a brick wall at about thirty-five miles. Thirty had become the new sixty.

Chapter Thirty-Three

By early April 2008, my ninety-day leave of absence from my job in New Jersey had been all but used up. There was one more stop to make before my return to employment: a trip down to Portland for my three-month checkup. I was feeling pretty good and was looking forward to seeing Dr. Daneshmand again, even though I was more than a little apprehensive about the visit, knowing that it would involve an invasive test.

So early on the morning of April 26th, Laura and I once again made the drive south from Sammamish, arriving at the OHSU clinic building, the Health and Wellness Center, before our 11:00 a.m. appointment. We proceeded to the lab, where ample quantities of blood and urine were collected. After a chest x-ray, we went up to the tenth floor to Urology. Chest x-rays had become a part of my regular testing, as the most common destination for distant bladder cancer metastasis is the lungs.

We were greeted warmly by Mark Johnson, who sat with us in the waiting lobby for a few minutes asking how I was doing. A short while later, after being weighed and blood-pressured, I was taken to an exam room, where Laura and I waited for the boss.

Dr. Daneshmand swept into the room with his trademark broad smile, and announced that I looked great. He wasted no time in reporting on the hematology and urinalysis, saying that everything was completely normal for three months out, and most importantly, there was no trace of any cancer cells anywhere.

He told me what came next: another cystogram. At the time of my first cystogram three months before, I still had the catheter in place from the surgery so it was a piece of cake. This time I would need to be catheterized, drained, and infused with a liquid that would provide contrast to get a clearer picture of the plumbing. I was apprehensive, of course, but had been told by Mark that 90% of the discomfort during catheterization was from the prostate. Mine had been removed during surgery, and I recalled that my brief period of self-catheterization had not been painful or even especially uncomfortable.

In went the pipe, and then the contrast. I did experience some discomfort as the neobladder stretched to capacity, but it was not really pain, more of a feeling of over-fullness. Then the machine was lowered over my lower abdomen and my insides appeared magically in full color on a high-definition flat screen over the bed. I was fascinated as Dr. Daneshmand showed me the ureters going from the kidneys into the neobladder and the way it was stretched into the old bladder cavity perfectly. He was very pleased with his work, and told me right away that there were no abnormalities and certainly no sign of tumors. He then drained the contrast, easily removed the catheter, and a nurse cleaned me up.

We had a fifteen-minute debriefing in his office. He inquired about continence, impotence, digestive system issues, and fatigue. I answered his questions as openly and honestly as I could, feeling no embarrassment or nervousness. He congratulated me on the speed of my recovery, particularly the early walking, a quick return to daytime continence, and the resumption of some kind of sex life.

It was a very happy trip back to Sammamish that afternoon after a celebratory late lunch in Portland.

BACK TO LIFE

Chapter Thirty-Four

Although fatigue was still an issue, it was time to gently re-engage, the first order of business being a return to work. I worked from home in Sammamish for the first week after my check-up, having some lengthy phone conversations with my boss to help me catch up with the goings-on at the company over the previous ninety days. I also reached out to an inner circle of friends in the industry, letting them know I was back in the game and not much worse for wear.

The following Monday morning at 5:15 a.m., a black town car pulled into the driveway of our home. I kissed Laura goodbye, put my roller bag in the trunk, threw my briefcase/backpack on the back seat, and jumped in. I was on the way to SeaTac airport, headed for the main office in New Jersey for two weeks.

It felt a bit strange getting back on the early morning 737

nonstop to Newark that I had taken so many times in the last year and a half. Settling into my seat, I wondered if I was trying too hard and coming back too soon. An hour later I had been fed breakfast and good strong coffee, and I settled into reading a mystery on my Kindle e-reader, feeling confident that I was doing the right thing.

In my backpack briefcase in the overhead was the road kit that Mark Johnson had assembled for me. It contained a sealed half-liter bottle of prescription saline solution, a sterile catheter, the turkey-baster injector, packets of lube, alcohol swabs, and hand sanitizer. Considering the long flight and extremely low humidity on airplanes, there was a constant danger of dehydration, which could easily cause the mucous in my neobladder to thicken to the point of forming a clog. That would not be a good thing at 33,000 feet! The idea was that if I were to experience an inability to urinate, I had everything I needed to irrigate and flush the neobladder in a safe and sterile fashion. I was drinking water pretty much nonstop to avoid this scary contingency.

We landed about four hours later at Newark Liberty International airport, where I was met by another town-car driver at baggage claim. He held the standard name sign, but when I looked more closely, it had a "Welcome Back" message before my name. I smiled broadly as I identified myself and let him know I had carried on my belongings. We walked to the parking lot and headed for Mahwah, New Jersey, some forty-five minutes away up NJ 17.

Since it made no sense for the company to keep paying for my old apartment for the months I had been gone, we had given it up and returned all the rented furniture and company-loaned electronics. I was to stay at the Mahwah Doubletree Hotel, just a short three-minute drive from our headquarters. I had stayed there before, when I interviewed for the job, and again when I first started with the company, plus it was one of two preferred spots for our overseas colleagues' stays when they came to Mahwah for big international meetings. So I knew it well. It was an aged, depressing hotel, with threadbare brown carpeting in the hallways and an ancient-looking bar and grill. The rooms had all been renovated, however, and the bedding was new. The place was also clean, if somewhat tired. Since the company did lots of business with this hotel and I was staying two weeks a month, I got a massive mini-suite with a sitting room, working desk, and two big flat-screen TVs.

Instead of taking me directly to the hotel, I asked the driver to take me to my storage unit, where I opened the garage-style door and retrieved my SUV. It was already after 4:00 p.m. and I knew I could just go check in at the hotel, but I went to the office instead, where I received a warm welcome from the executives on my floor and a tearful hug from my assistant, Michele. I walked into my office, took my notebook computer out of my backpack, slid it into the docking station, and sat down behind my big desk.

I was back.

Chapter Thirty-Five

My first two-week stint back in New Jersey passed quickly. I was in the office early every morning, but left shortly after 5:00 each afternoon, bone tired. I had dinner most nights at the bar in the hotel's restaurant, but every few nights I'd need a change and walked down to a local bar and grill called the Mason Jar. It was full of very friendly locals, and I soon became known to both the wait staff and most of the regular patrons. The food was simple but good, and a cut above the hotel food.

I remained very fatigued, and fell into bed early most nights after an hour or so of TV or reading. My spirits remained high, however, and I quickly settled into a work rhythm, albeit at a somewhat slower pace than before the surgery. The second Friday flight home could not come soon enough.

I had a noon flight out of Newark nonstop to Seattle, so I left the office about 9:30 a.m., drove to the airport, and sought out the long-term parking lot. Heading through security at EWR, I experienced the first of what would be many terrible experiences with the TSA folks. I had done my research on their policy for carry-on medications, and up to a half liter of prescription saline was specifically called out as approved on the TSA Web site. As a precaution, I carried both a printout of that Web page and a laminated, signed letter from Dr. Daneshmand attesting to the necessity of my carrying the road kit, including the sealed sterile saline.

In accordance with the TSA instructions, I removed my kit, which was housed in a clear gallon baggie, placed it in a bin along with my toiletries, and announced to the screener that I was carrying a medical kit. He responded with a grunt. As my belongings came out on the other side, he called for a supervisor to look at my kit. This is exactly what had happened two weeks before in Seattle, where they knew their rules. They simply swabbed the outside of the bottle, cleared the swab through their detecting device, and had me on my way in less than two minutes with a polite thank you.

New Jersey proved a bit different, to say the least. The supervisor sauntered over about five minutes later and read the label on the bottle.

"Sodium chloride," he said, eyebrows raised, in a deepened voice that could have been saying "nitroglycerin."

"It's prescription saline solution," I said. "Salt water."

I should have shut up right then, but I went on. "It's specifically permitted according to the TSA Web site. Here, I have a printout of the Web page."

"Anybody can put anything on a Web page and print it," he said in a confrontational tone. He was right, of course.

"I also have a letter from my urologist explaining why I need to carry it on."

His frown deepened. "I don't need a letter from anybody," he said. "I just need to open it up and test it."

"You can't do that!" I said, just a little too urgently. His bearing visibly stiffened.

"You're not the one deciding what we do or don't do."

I realized we were heading down a bad road here, so I softened my tone, held my arms out in a gesture of surrender, and said, "Please let me explain, sir. In an emergency, the saline solution has to go into my body through a catheter, which is right there in the bag. The saline has got to be sterile, and opening it up could contaminate it and make it useless to me." He grunted and walked off carrying my kit without a word.

He returned in about ten minutes with *his* supervisor, and we did the whole dance over from the beginning. They both retreated to an office, where I assume they looked at their own Web site, because when they returned they handed me my kit and walked away without so much as an apology. The worst part of it was that after nearly a half hour of going around in circles, *they never even tested the outside of the bottle.* I could see the exact same testing equipment used in Seattle not ten feet away.

The bottom line is I *could* have had a bottle of nitroglycerin and they would never have known. I have been through many, many similar fiascos, usually in small airports like Burbank, California, but Newark has consistently been the very worst.

An uneventful flight followed, and I exited security in Seattle to find my wife waiting for me. It was great to be home.

Chapter Thirty-Six

There were important planning meetings for the company's European region starting in a week's time, so the plan was for me to rest up for a week working from home, then head out on my first international trip since my return. I would fly nonstop to Amsterdam from Seattle and take the fifty-minute train ride from Schiphol airport to Eindhoven, the home of our EU headquarters.

I was to fly out Saturday afternoon. The flight was just under ten hours to Amsterdam, and with that and the time difference, I would land at about 8:00 on Sunday morning. I had some apprehension about the length of the flight and the nine-hour time difference, due to the still persistent fatigue, but overall I was in fine spirits and looking forward to getting back to Europe.

I had no idea that I was approaching the most embarrassing moments of my life.

Laura dropped me off at SeaTac airport at noon on Saturday, and I checked my roller-bag and headed through security. The Seattle TSA crew tested my saline bottle efficiently and once again politely sent on my way. As I settled into my uncomfortable business-class seat on the huge Airbus A330, I felt confident that with proper rest and diet I could handle the six-day trip without issue.

The flight was long and uneventful. I read a book by one of my favorite authors, Robert Crais, on my trusty Kindle, had a decent dinner, and rested my eyes for a while with some music on the iPod. After over eight hours of flight, we began our slow descent over the English Channel.

I never sleep on airplanes. Sure, I doze a bit, but I really never go fully into sleep. Perhaps it was the lingering fatigue from my cancer surgery, or maybe it was the first really long flight I'd been on in almost a half a year, but about forty-five minutes out from landing, I fell sound asleep.

I woke up about five minutes later and immediately realized I had released my bladder. I was pissing my pants! I clamped down on the urinary sphincter and immediately stopped the flow, but the damage had been done. A large dark stain covered my crotch and went halfway down my left leg. I was mortified. I had been sitting in an aisle seat to the left of the left aisle, with one person next to me in the window seat. He was staring at the growing stain.

There's one thing I haven't had occasion to mention until now. For the first year or more, urine from a neobladder smells terrible in addition to being full of mucous. It kind of makes sense when you consider that it was built from a section of intestine. In any case, there I sat, soaking wet and smelling pretty awful. And there was very little I could do about it. Changing was out of the question, as my bag had been checked.

I got up quickly because I knew we were minutes from seat-belt time, and I headed for the rest room. There I tried my best to soak up as much as I could with paper towels on the inside of my jeans and underwear, and washed myself off with soap and warm water. Then I returned to my seat and apologized to my seatmate.

"Did you have too much to drink?" he asked. He had been sleeping for most of the night, so he couldn't know that I had nothing but water.

"No, actually I've had no alcohol at all."

So I explained that I had had fairly recent surgery for bladder cancer and that it was natural to leak some while sleeping, and also that I typically never fall asleep during flights. I also explained the smell in layman's terms, and he seemed less aggravated after learning I wasn't some drunk. We started our final approach into Schiphol airport, and I dreaded what I knew was coming.

As I was in business class relatively close to the front of the plane, I was, blessedly, able to exit the plane quickly and head for immigration control. Unfortunately, at that time of the morning there were several other jumbo jets that had made overnight crossings of the Atlantic from various North American cities. So there were several hundred people in front of me, and in my mind every single one of them was staring at my pee-stained jeans.

I was exhausted and depressed as I finally cleared immigration and headed out to the baggage claim. Luckily, my bag was one of the first ones to come down the chute. Next came customs, where I received disapproving stares from the officials. Or maybe they were looks of pity. In any case, I walked through without being stopped. Another bit of good fortune was the airport at which I had landed. Schiphol is one of the most modern and best-appointed airports in the world, and as such has coin-operated showers in the rest rooms.

I peeled off my clothes, inserted a couple of euros, and washed away the embarrassment with a handful of strong Dutch soap. I dried myself with a clean t-shirt from my bag and put on clean clothes. I had only brought one pair of jeans, so I changed into dress slacks and a clean shirt. Not the most stylish ensemble but about a million percent improvement over peed-in jeans. The jeans, underwear, and t-shirt went in the trashcan in the rest room, as I had no plastic bag to keep them from contaminating the rest of the clothes. Plus that smell.

My ordeal finally over, I bought a train ticket and headed down the escalator in the main terminal hall to the tracks, where I caught a train for the quick trip to Eindhoven.

The meetings that week went smoothly, and I felt in great shape except for the persistent fatigue. But I was learning to cope with it. There's one term you hear frequently from folks who have had cancer treatments, surgery in particular. It's "the new normal," and refers to adjusting one's attitude to accept that things will not return to the way they were. I felt I was making good progress accepting my own new normal of fatigue and occasional nighttime incontinence, carefully watching my diet and particularly my evening fluid intake.

I flew home on Friday after the quick morning train ride back to Schiphol. Needless to say, there was a spare adult absorbency product in my briefcase! Flying east to west, we were picking up eight hours, so the flight landed the same afternoon in Seattle. I was never close to sleep throughout the ten-and-a-half-hour flight back. I was definitely glad to be home, met at the airport by my wonderful wife. We both had tears in our eyes as we embraced at baggage claim.

Chapter Thirty-Seven

Spring eased into summer, and I fell back into my travel routine, spending two weeks per month at the lovely Mahwah Doubletree. In June I made my first trip back to Japan, visiting our headquarters in Yokohama, not far from Tokyo. It was on this trip that I first realized the stigma that is attached to cancer in most of the world.

I had not yet encountered any of this, as I had only been among close friends and business associates in the USA, and only in the Netherlands on my one trip to Europe. I have found the Dutch to be some of the most intelligent, respectful, and empathetic people in the world, and those at the company who knew my story never treated me the slightest bit differently after my return.

My experience in Japan was quite different. While my American counterparts were just fine, most of the Japanese who had heard about my illness would not even look at me.

A couple of my closer Japanese associates made an effort to act normal, but it was obvious that it was taking some effort, which was in itself very awkward. I was never again treated as I was before my illness, and it upset me quite a lot, especially as it was so totally unexpected.

We've come a long way in the United States, thanks to the pink ribbons, the Lance Armstrong Foundation (now Livestrong,) and many other well-meaning organizations. Even today in rural Africa, those afflicted with cancer are routinely driven out of their villages and left to suffer and die alone. But major stigma still exists in First World, post-industrial countries like Italy, where it is taboo to talk about cancer, and cancer in a family is considered a deep dishonor. It exists here too, if in a lesser form. Exactly 100% of the people I've spoken to who are living with and through cancer and its aftermath have told of friends who have simply vanished permanently from their lives, apparently unable to deal with the reality of cancer so close at hand. Regrettably, I have experienced this myself, having lost quite a few long-time close friends suddenly and completely. All of this behavior does a great disservice to the cancer survivor. The psychological burdens of the post-cancer life are many, and to be looked at strangely and whispered about is just about the worst feeling you can imagine. The pain of having friends vanish suddenly, inexplicably, and permanently is devastating. Throw in the inevitable survivors' guilt that we all feel, and you have recipe for sadness, depression, and worse.

The vocabulary of those writing about cancer is dripping with comparisons to war. Nobody dies from cancer; they "lost their courageous battle." Almost everyone I have spoken with in the cancer community hates this. As one of my favorite cancer wits put it: "When someone dies in a car accident, you never hear about how they lost their brave battle with a Subaru."

Many of the folks I have spoken with are deeply uncomfortable with the whole "survivor" terminology. To many, it demeans those who die from cancer, and let's face it, more people die from cancer than are cured. It seems like you are self-identifying as somehow superior, when all of us know how fortunate we are to be among the minority whose treatment has worked, if only for now. We're surviving, I suppose, but does that make us survivors? And if we're not survivors, then what *do* we call ourselves? I've not yet heard the perfect name, and I don't think there really is one, but a cancer friend likes to call us "veterans." I must say I like all of the connotations of that word in relation to cancer, even though it does have the old war overtones. I've run this one by many cancer—ahem—veterans, and most seem more comfortable with this term than others.

Chapter Thirty-Eight

In early June, I composed my annual fundraising letter for the 2008 Ride for the Roses. I sent it via email and snail mail to over two hundred family members, friends, business colleagues, and acquaintances. I wrote a bit about returning from cancer and the symbolic importance of literally and figuratively getting "back in the saddle." I also said in my appeal that this would be the last time I asked for their support. Not that I wouldn't ever attend the Ride for the Roses again, but I pledged to fund it personally rather than solicit their contributions.

This was a strategic move. In 2008 the country was in the depths of recession, and I knew that raising money would be more difficult than in any of my four prior campaigns. My thought was that people would dig just a bit deeper knowing they were not going to get hit on again year after year for money. I had ridden the Austin ride for four consecutive years, from 2003 through 2006, and I had achieved the coveted "Yellow Jersey Team" status each year.

To make the fundraising process more fun—and competitive—the Foundation issued four fundraising levels each year, which were named after the four primary jerseys of the Tour de France. From lowest to highest, they were: the White Jersey Team, named for the best young rider's jersey; the Green Jersey Team, referring to the jersey awarded to the best points rider, typically the best sprinter; the Polka Dot Jersey Team, after the jersey of the king of the mountains or best climber; and of course the Yellow Jersey Team, named for the overall race leader's jersey.

The Yellow Jersey Team was composed of those whose fundraising results had exceeded the top fundraising target. Each year there were approximately thirty to forty riders that achieved Yellow Jersey Team status and the attending perks, which were very significant in addition to the pride of accomplishment. First, the Foundation picked up the round-trip airfare to Austin, the bike transportation charge ($75 each way), the hotel room for three nights, and most meals. All this for both the fundraiser and his or her guest—in my case Laura. In addition, there was a private Friday-night cocktail party for the Yellow Jersey Team at a cool location, attended by Lance Armstrong and many of his celebrity friends, including, on our previous three trips, Sheryl Crow, Robin Williams, Will Farrell, Lyle Lovett, and many of Lance's teammates on the US Postal Service Team. Then Saturday afternoon the Yellow and Polka Dot teams assembled outside the hotel, where they were whisked away in buses to a secret location outside of town. Upon arrival, we noticed that our bikes had been carefully wrapped in movers' blankets and trucked out to the site, where they were carefully lined up in huge bike racks. There was even a complete bike repair shop set up at the start/finish line. Yes, this was the granddaddy of all perks: a private ride with Lance.

Saturday night, before the big ride on Sunday, there was the annual banquet dinner at another cool location—this one for the Green, Polka Dot, and Yellow teams, which totaled several hundred people. There were games, mechanical bull rides, and a huge silent auction that included autographed guitars, rare vintage bicycles, and even private rides with some of Lance's more famous teammates like George Hincapie.

If all this seems a bit extravagant if not downright financially irresponsible for a charity organization, remember that the ride raises millions of dollars each year, and the thirty odd Yellow Jersey Team members raise an average of over $80,000 each annually.

Chapter Thirty-Nine

Through the rest of the summer of 2008 and into September, I tried to log as many miles as possible, but with the extensive travel and lingering fatigue I had only ridden just over a thousand miles by the end of September. That may sound like a lot, but in my cycling prime I would log well over three thousand miles before the Ride for the Roses, and at a much more athletic pace and over tougher terrain. I was getting worried about even being fit enough to complete the one-hundred-kilometer (sixty-two-mile) course I had signed up for.

The fundraising was also not going well. The recession had put even more of a damper than I had expected on the generosity quotient, and to compound the issue the Foundation had set the highest fundraising bar ever for the Yellow Jersey Team.

I was in New Jersey for the first two weeks of October, and tried my best to hit the stationary bike in the hotel exercise room for an hour every day after work in an attempt to at least maintain whatever level of fitness I had managed to attain. After returning from New Jersey, I went for a cold, rainy ride on Saturday morning, October 11th, just thirteen days before our departure for Austin. The cold rain, the jet travel all day on Friday, and my lack of real saddle time over the previous two weeks were the proverbial perfect storm, and I cracked badly after about twenty-five miles, still nine miles from home. My route ended with a one-mile climb at a nine-degree gradient, which is very steep. When I approached it I was near tears. Was there any chance at all that I could ride a hundred kilometers just two weeks hence?

It was the biggest crisis in confidence I had experienced since the pipes were removed in February. I rode the final climb at barely 5 mph, about half my pre-cancer pace, just fast enough to stay upright. I was in a foul mood at the dinner table that night and not very good company at all.

After a good night's sleep and some strong Seattle coffee, my outlook improved the following morning. It was still raining, so I headed to the gym instead of venturing out for another ride. Lots of stretching, an hour of spinning, and some light leg work with the weight machines left me tired, but in a good way. Add a healthy dinner cooked at home, and I wound up with a big bounce back from my mini-crisis.

I rode almost every day for the following week and a half. The weather cooperated with unseasonably warm temperatures and only a couple days with light rain. The Sunday before we left for Austin was sunny and cool, and Jeff and I knocked out a brisk forty miles, even including the gentle (4% average gradient) three-mile climb up the back side of Ames Lake Road over the Tolt Ridge.

It was also the deadline to qualify for the various jersey teams. I had put out a final appeal in mid-September asking for additional contributions, but the well was dry. I received less than a thousand dollars more from that final appeal, and still fell many thousands short of the Yellow Jersey quota. I realized how important being on that team was to me as a cancer veteran. After a discussion with Laura, I logged on to my donation page and made a large anonymous donation to the Foundation that put me $50 over the Yellow Jersey amount.

Finally it was time, and I packed my prized Trek Madone into its hard-shell airline case, and checked for extra tubes, chain lube, cycling shorts, jerseys, arm and leg warmers, and a rain jacket. We headed to the SeaTac airport on Friday morning, October 24th, for our flight to Dallas/Fort Worth and on to Austin.

Chapter Forty

There was a buzz in the air at the airport as flights from around the country delivered the riders to Austin. The oversized luggage chutes were disgorging bike cases of all sizes and shapes, most with colorful identifying stickers because there were many identical cases. We quickly located my bike and headed to the Livestrong desk, where we were welcomed as Yellow Jersey Team members and directed to the waiting bus.

The lobby of the Embassy Suites was humming with energy, and we were directed to the VIP bike-assembly room, where Trek mechanics expertly—and very deftly—assembled my bike, tuned it up, and deposited it in a secure lockup along with its case. After checking in and grabbing a coffee in the lobby, we began to see folks we knew from previous years arriving at the hotel. This is always one of the most heartrending moments of the trip, because there are always people missing. It's a young husband back this year as a widower, a young couple who were here two years ago with their ten-year-old daughter, and are now childless. The reality of cancer puts a somber backdrop behind the weekend's camaraderie and festivities.

At 6 p.m. we headed over to the convention center, where the Yellow Jersey cocktail party was to begin. What in years past had been one of the two best perks of being in Yellow turned out to be the most disappointing part of the whole weekend. The party was held in a totally generic, nondescript meeting room with a small open bar at one end. The only "celebrity" to attend was the Japanese president of Shimano, the company that made the components for the US Postal Service Team's Trek bikes. A nice-enough guy who spoke a little heavily accented English, but not exactly Will Farrell! The Yellow Jersey fundraisers milled about uncertainly, waiting for Lance's celebrity friends to make an appearance. The party wound down after less than an hour, as the realization hit us all—no celebrities, no famous teammates, and worst of all, no Lance.

On Saturday we slept in and had a leisurely breakfast in the hotel restaurant. There was palpable electricity in the air among the Yellow and Polka-Dot teams, as this was the day of the ultimate perk, the private ride with Lance. Our bikes had been packed up and trucked to the secret location, and we gathered at noon in the hotel lobby, many of us sporting yellow and polka-dot jerseys from past years. It was about a forty-minute ride out to the start of the ride, and conversation on the bus was lively with excitement.

The weather was perfect, sunny and warm, and we arrived

to find the bikes lined up in racks. Like in past years there was a fully equipped Trek-staffed mobile bike-repair kiosk. We quickly located our rides and milled around waiting for the start of the show. While we waited, Laura and I said hi to our friend Liz Kreutz, the world-famous sports photographer who hails from Austin and is one of Lance's oldest friends. She has taken some terrific photos of not only cycling, but many other events over the years. Today she would be sitting in the back of the pace car, a convertible, photographing each team member's brief opportunity to ride "on the front" alone with Lance.

Just a few minutes later, Lance screamed up on his US Postal Service Trek Madone, accompanied by the members of a local cycling club that would serve as the "chaperones," directing traffic and guiding the riders to the front for their moment of glory. I walked over to Lance and said hello. He smiled, and then immediately changed to a mock frown.

"So where the hell were you last year?"

"I was busy."

"Too busy to come to Austin for the ride?" he said with a slight sneer.

"I had cancer," I said.

At that moment everything changed. He waved the other approaching riders off and we walked a few steps away.

"What was it?" he asked. "And is it out of you? How are you now?"

I told him what it was and gave the briefest possible explanation of the surgery.

"Holy shit," he said. "We'll talk more on the road."

The day could not have been more pleasant—about seventy-five degrees with a nice breeze. We rolled out behind the pace car corralled by a half dozen club members and turned out of the parking lot onto the road. The Foundation has learned a lot about how to conduct these rides over the years. For the first couple of years there was no pace car and no guide riders, so it was a complete free-for-all. Lance rode quickly to keep from getting mobbed, and all but the fittest cyclists were left behind in just a few minutes. Needless to say this did not sit well for the fundraisers who had spent months raising tens of thousands of dollars only to see Lance for a minute or so at the start.

After a couple of years of this chaos, the Foundation staff realized that just because someone raises a lot of money doesn't mean they are a competitive rider. We had women in their sixties on hybrid bikes who had no chance of staying with a fast-moving pack. I believe 2005 was the first year with a pace car and a rider rotation plan, and that was the answer. We rode about ten miles at about 12 mph, a leisurely pace indeed.

I did get a chance to speak with Lance a bit more during my turn on the front. He twice waved off the guide rider who was trying to bring up the next rider, and I finally said it was time for me to drop back. The last thing he said to me was, "If you need anything, if there is anything the Foundation can do to help you, you call, you hear?"

The rest of the ride went great, and afterwards we were treated to a catered lunch in a large meeting room at the facility that hosted the start/finish. Soon we were on the bus back to the hotel, where we would clean up, rest a bit, and then get ready for the long drive out to the big Saturday night dinner, which included the Green Jersey Team in addition to the Yellow and Polka Dot teams. This would bring the total attendance to almost two hundred. Spirits on the bus were soaring, and it seemed that everyone was satisfied with the highly organized, fair manner in which the private ride was managed.

After showers, a brief rest, and some more coffee with old friends down in the lobby, we got ready for the long bus ride out to a famous Texas barbecue spot. As the buses snaked down Colorado Street in Austin's downtown, we noticed the marquee of one of the many live-music venues proclaiming "Tonight Only — Marc Broussard." Marc Broussard was one of our favorite musicians, having written and played a song called "Home" on his first album that we first heard on the radio. It is a ferocious piece of Louisiana swamp rock that builds to an almost painfully intense musical climax. I remember thinking, "What if we just skipped the long bus ride to the Livestrong dinner and went to a show?" Little did I know what a good choice that would have been.

The traffic on the way out of Austin was brutal, and what had been promised as a forty-five minute bus ride stretched to over double that. It was dusk when we pulled up to the barbecue joint, an enormous place that was well equipped for large events. The food was served buffet-style, and was mediocre at best, another big disappointment. Lance gave an uncharacteristically brief and unfocused speech, thanking everyone for their support. We saw him only intermittently for the rest of the night.

The musical guest—musical entertainment being a regular occurrence at the big dinners—was Willie Nelson and his band. He's a long-term friend of Lance's, and we were all looking forward to his set. They were to play on a small stage in back of the big main building where we had eaten dinner. As it turned out, he and his band arrived in a fog of marijuana smoke and played so poorly that a half hour into their set there were fewer than fifty people listening. Most had drifted off, and some were already asking about early buses back to the hotel. We wished we had stayed in Austin for Marc Broussard!

All of this was doubly disappointing because the previous years' events had been fantastic. By far the best was in 2004, where the dinner was held at a wild game preserve located somewhat perversely behind the largest landfill in the Texas Hill Country. There were rides, roping demonstrations, and roving singing cowboys outside on the lawns as the sun began to set. A large silent auction was in full swing. Inside the main building was a beautiful hall where a full sit-down dinner was served. The Yellow Jersey Team members were seated at four tables front and center, and Laura and I were sitting back-to-back with Lance and Sheryl Crow! Laura had her camera, and I grabbed the opportunity to ask Sheryl for a picture together. Although she has a reputation as somewhat of a diva, this night she could not have been nicer.

Lance gave an impassioned speech about the Foundation's mission, and he closed his talk with a statement he would make many times thereafter.

"I have one wish, and that's to live long enough to raise a glass with all of you and say 'Can you believe we actually once used to give people chemotherapy?'"

Laura got a chance to meet Robin Williams up close and

personal, and she treasures those brief moments to this day, particularly in light of his tragic suicide. After dinner, we retired to the natural outdoor amphitheater behind the building, where a stage had been erected.

We were treated to one of the flat-out funniest—if also one of the flat-out dirtiest—improvised standup routines ever, courtesy of the aforementioned Mr. Williams. He riffed on all of the animals in the game preserve, giving each a unique personality, many of which were some of his standard impressions, like the Galois-puffing Frenchman.

This was followed by an incredible solo acoustic set by Sheryl Crow. Lance joined her to sing off-key backup vocals on her last song, and was greeted by good-natured calls of "Don't quit your day job!" from friends in the audience.

Compared to that memorable night, the 2008 dinner was sadly lacking.

Chapter Forty-One

It was still pitch dark the next morning as the riders drifted into the hotel lobby. There was a special cash buffet set up there that offered coffee, juices, yogurt, bagels, and fruit. I loaded up on a cinnamon raisin bagel with cream cheese, two bananas, and copious amounts of black coffee. In front of the hotel, steam poured out of the buses' exhausts in the cold, dark Texas morning.

It was about a forty-five minute drive out to the big school complex that would serve as the start/finish line and the site of the post-ride party, which featured live bands as well as plenty of food and drink, cookout style. The conversation on the bus was subdued, with most riders chatting quietly with their partners. We were all thinking about the physical challenge to come, and no one more so than yours truly.

The weather in the Texas Hill Country in October is nothing if not unpredictable. The pre-dawn temperatures can be in the low forties at the beginning of the ride, and it can easily hit the high nineties by the noontime finish. One year it was in the high thirties at the start, with many riders clad in nothing but cycling shorts and a short-sleeve jersey. That year I was shaking so hard at the start that I thought I might crash, but I had at least thought to stuff a pair of fleece arm warmers in my back pocket.

On Sunday, October 26th, 2008, the day started out cool and clear, with just a light breeze blowing, near ideal conditions for a long ride. I proudly rolled out with the first group, which included Lance and his group of celebrity friends followed by the different jersey teams in order. My strategy was the same as in past years: try to find a large group of experienced riders that were going at a comfortable pace for me to hang in with. I had no illusions that this was going to be anything like the screaming-fast rides of years past.

As I tried to hang with one group, then another and another, I realized that even my modest expectations were too optimistic. I finally settled in with my fourth or fifth group, riding on the mainly flat first part of the course at barely 15 mph.

A little under two hours into the ride I pulled off the group at the twenty-five-mile rest stop. I needed some nutrition and refills on my water and energy-drink bottles. I ate a banana and some wheat bread slathered with peanut butter, stretched a bit, and pulled out after barely a ten-minute stop, trying to avoid the muscle tightness that comes with longer breaks out of the saddle.

About three miles down the road, struggling to stay with yet another group going around 15 mph, I began to feel light-headed and nauseous. I knew this was not good, particularly as I had not yet made it to the halfway point of the hundred-kilometer ride, the thirty-one-mile mark. I soldiered on, getting dropped by one group after another, and finally, almost three and a half hours after starting, I pulled into the forty-five-mile rest stop. I had serious doubts as to whether I would or could remount the bike.

I stayed at the rest stop way too long. After drinking water, refilling my bottles, and eating a Cliff bar that tasted like peanut butter mixed with sawdust, I lay down on my back in the shade of a fence along side the road. I remember looking up at the puffy white clouds and the cobalt blue Texas sky. I have no idea how long I lay there, but when I stood up I was dizzy and disoriented and my legs were stiff and sore. The bus that was parked there to take abandoning riders back to the start/finish area beckoned. The sun was high in the cloudless sky and the temperature broke ninety degrees. I had seventeen more miles to go.

When you do the Ride for the Roses, the Foundation provides you with a rider number for your jersey, but also offers three different placards to attach to your jersey or bike. The first two are "In Honor Of..." and "In Memory Of... ." You write in the name of your friend, relative, or loved one who has survived cancer or who has been killed by it. The third sign simply says, "I Am a Cancer Survivor." My past four rides, I had worn the first two, one for my cancer-veteran wife and one for my good friend's wife who died from breast cancer. It was her death that motivated me to raise well over a quarter of a million dollars for the Foundation over the course of my five rides.

In 2008 I had a fourth sign on my back in addition to the race number and the two memorials. *I am a cancer survivor.* I thought about that fourth sign as I contemplated the alternatives: walk across the grass in front of the rest stop and put my bike in the bus and climb aboard, or throw a leg over it and give it one more try. With the words "In Honor Of…" and "In Memory Of…" singing in my head, the decision was easy. I rode unsteadily out onto the course, legs stiff and achy, stomach churning, head pounding under the noonday sun.

After the first two miles, I was questioning my decision. People on hybrids and mountain bikes who in past years would have finished the better part of two hours behind me were cruising up and passing. With my carbon-fiber bike and full Livestrong Yellow Jersey Team kit, it was obvious that this was a rider in distress.

Then a strange thing happened. As a small group approached me, they began to call out, encouraging me to keep on riding. I realized that it was the survivor badge pinned to the back of my jersey. I waved and smiled, and five minutes later it happened again, and then again.

I still had twelve miles to go, and I remembered one of the mental tricks we used to use when we were suffering at the end of long rides. We would say to ourselves, "I can survive anything for ten miles." So the goal became the ten-mile mark rather than the finish line. It sounds like a pretty cheesy motivator, but it actually had worked for my friends and me more than once. I said it out loud: "I have only two miles to go. Then I can survive anything for ten miles!"

With about five miles left, I heard the unmistakable

thrum of aerodynamic racing wheels; a large group of fast riders was approaching. It was a group about to complete the 108-mile route that I had done in previous years, and they had nearly doubled my speed to be passing me. I pulled far to the right as they approached.

It was a group of about thirty guys, and as they flew by me I noticed several polka-dot jerseys and a couple of yellows. Then I heard a shout, "Hey, I think that's Frank!"

Suddenly two riders dropped off the back of the group and slowed quickly. They drifted back to where I was huffing along at about 11 or 12 mph. It was two of my Yellow Jersey cronies with whom I had ridden in several of the rides over the years.

"Jesus, dude, are you OK?" said Jim, who was a forty-something doctor from Texas and a very strong rider. Both of them were looking at me with clear concern.

"Thanks guys," I said, "but I'm totally toast. I'm just going to ride my own pace on in. I'll be OK. No need for you two to wait around. Ride on."

"Fuck we will," said David, an investment counselor from Montana. "Hop on."

In cycling terms, they were offering to pace me in to the finish, allowing me to ride in their slipstream and conserve valuable energy. They ignored my pleas for them to leave me, and rode together very closely side by side in order to give me the maximum benefit of their draft. It is gesture of camaraderie and compassion that I will never forget.

The finish line at the Ride for the Roses is unlike any other. The approach road is lined with hundreds of cheering spectators, volunteers, and friends and relatives of the riders.

As you approach the line, the route divides in two; the smaller lane on the left is just for cancer survivors, while the larger lane to the right is for everybody else, the "civilians" as the volunteer ride marshals called them.

Laura had warned me about this. A few years back she had done one of the shorter rides while I did the big one, and she, as a survivor, naturally went through the appropriate lane, where she was handed the traditional yellow rose. I was still out on the course at the time, but she described the flood of emotions that overtook her when she crossed the line and accepted the rose. Naturally, I told her that was unlikely to be a problem for me. After all, I'm a big tough guy, right?

Yeah, right.

The last three hundred meters of the course ascended a small rise to the finishing straight. My two protectors pulled away with a wave as they delivered me to the split in the course. They were going right, but I was going to the left. I had been woozy and mentally and physically sluggish for several hours, but in those last few moments before crossing the line everything was crystal clear. I heard every cheer of encouragement, saw every waving flag. And then the banner was upon me. Under I went, too exhausted to even raise my arms in the traditional cyclist's finishing salute. I coasted up to the volunteer who extended her hand with a single yellow rose.

I took the rose and coasted slowly over to the side, away from the finishers swooping through the chute. I saw Laura standing there with tears in her eyes. I dropped my bike on the ground and we wrapped our arms around each other. And then I totally lost it, literally crying on her shoulder for many minutes.

Chapter Forty-Two

We walked my bike to the lock-up area and went out to the post-ride party that was in full swing, with a band playing on a huge stage, and food and drink stalls all around. We had missed Lance's brief speech, of course, since I finished hours behind his group.

I remember drinking a cold Coke and trying to eat a hamburger, but it was not party time for me. We gave up after about a half hour and made our way to the buses, where the first wave was getting ready to depart. We retrieved my bike and stowed it in the luggage area of the bus.

I really don't remember the ride back or getting to the hotel, but after a long hot shower and some fluids, I actually felt much better. I tried to rationalize my perceived failure and to celebrate that I had in fact accomplished my main goal of riding the one-hundred-kilometer course. It wasn't working, so I tried to push it out of my mind and concentrate on the rest of our evening, for Laura's sake if not my own.

You would think Austin, Texas, is about the last place on earth to find great Japanese food, but in fact Austin boasts not one, but two excellent sushi joints. We went to Uchi, not far from our hotel, and had a fantastic authentic Japanese dinner, with excellent sashimi and sushi. The highlight of the dinner was the "Wagyu Hot Rock," a dish seldom seen in Japanese restaurants in the US. They bring you a river rock, a large smooth pebble-shaped stone about five inches across, which has been heated to glowing. You get a plate of thick-sliced Wagyu beef tenderloin and a bowl of Ponzu sauce, and cook the beef yourself—in seconds—on the sizzling hot rock. A wonderful meal to be sure, and a great end to our Austin trip.

Chapter Forty-Three

With our return from Austin in October 2008, my bladder cancer story begins to wind down. I was incredibly discouraged by my performance on the ride, and I did not get back on the bike for several weeks. The holidays felt surprisingly empty to me that year, which I attributed to my poor fitness and a good dose of the aforementioned survivors' guilt, which is definitely a real thing for most cancer survivors.

I traveled to Portland in late January 2009 for my one-year follow up at OHSU with Dr. Daneshmand. Following morning labs and the usual chest x-ray, he performed another cystogram to look at the neobladder and pronounced it one of his best efforts. He enthusiastically pointed out how the bladder had formed itself into the cavity where my natural bladder had been, even stating that only a trained urologist would even be able to tell that it was not my natural bladder.

That amazed me. The best news was that there was no evidence whatsoever of any recurrence of cancer.

I had been reading everything I could find about neobladder surgery, and one of the things I remembered to ask Dr. Daneshmand about was neobladder surgery in women. Although women are much less likely to be diagnosed with bladder cancer, they are far less likely to have the neobladder as their urinary diversion. From Dr. Daneshmand I learned that the majority of surgeons were reluctant to use neobladders with women due the their unique physiology, particularly post-childbirth pelvic-floor weakness, which makes continence much more challenging with the neobladder. Also, approximately 30% of female neobladder recipients need ongoing regular catheterization versus just 10% of men. Even so, Dr. Daneshmand was frankly critical of the surgeons who refuse to learn effective surgical techniques unique to women's challenges, and he performs a higher percentage of neobladders on women than anyone.

He set my next appointment for six months out instead of ninety days, and I felt somewhat better on the long ride home.

As the rainy months commenced in the Seattle suburbs, my mood took a darker turn, and by February 2009 I knew something was wrong. I simply could not shake the deep sense of failure I took home from the Austin ride a few months prior. I probably should have been proud to even complete the ride so soon after my illness, but the reality was actually the opposite. What had been a kind of vague unease was blossoming into full-blown depression. I read a lot about the symptoms, and when I read that many sufferers of depression describe it as an almost physical weight bearing down upon them, I knew they were describing exactly what I was feeling. Nightly, my dreams were filled with a crushing sadness, and daily I awakened emotionally drained and physically exhausted.

I made an appointment with my primary care physician, and she concurred that the symptoms I was describing were those of classic depression. She congratulated me for coming in and trying to deal with it, as many people either can't or won't recognize that they have a mental health problem. She wanted to put me on an antidepressant drug, and I pushed back, having read that most of these drugs depress the libido. I was not joking when I said, "As hard as I've worked to regain sexual function, something that hinders my progress is going to make me *really* depressed."

She recommended that I go to a psychological counselor before we tried drugs. This was a disaster, and the less said about it the better. The guy I spoke to basically told me I had nothing to be depressed about, questioned that I was in fact depressed at all, and cavalierly gave me a photocopied article about the benefits of probiotics in maintaining mental health. I would have been even more depressed if I hadn't been so pissed off.

When I returned to my doctor's office, she had the answer in an antidepressant drug that not only did not lower the sex drive but was actually used to enhance it in some patients. I started taking this drug, called Wellbutrin, in March 2009. It helped me almost immediately.

Chapter Forty-Four

As the weather began to improve in late spring, I returned to the bike, mostly thanks to Jeff showing up and hauling me out. By mid-summer I was riding forty-milers regularly and even ascending some of our old climbs. The drug was working. The depression had receded, and I was in good spirits for the first time in ages. I had resigned my executive position and was no longer commuting to New Jersey, nor was I jetting off to Europe or Asia for a week every month.

Laura and I had been looking at condos, both in Seattle and Portland, with a view to downsizing our life now that our youngest was halfway through college and seldom home. We chose Portland because we loved the downtown in general and a planned mixed-use neighborhood called the Pearl District in particular. We bought a condo there in September, and after spending two months plus as tax exiles in our Las Vegas condo, we permanently relocated to Portland in November.

One of the many great features of Portland life is the fantastic public transportation system, which includes the first new downtown streetcar system built in a US city in over thirty years. There was a streetcar stop a block from our new home, and it went all the way through town, ending at the OHSU clinic building, which is where I went for my now annual checkups.

We enjoyed our first downsized Christmas and New Year's and after a week in Las Vegas for the annual Consumer Electronics Show, we rode the streetcar to OHSU for my annual visit with Dr. Daneshmand. It was purely routine and all the tests were once again 100% negative for any trace of a cancer recurrence.

At the end of the afternoon we met briefly with Dr. Daneshmand to recap the test results and answer all of his questions about my health and my perceived quality of life. It was then that we told him of our move to Portland, and our intention of riding the streetcar down to see him for many years to come.

Then he dropped the bombshell.

"I'm leaving OHSU in a couple of months," he said. "My wife and I are moving back to the Los Angeles area, which is where we're from and where I did my residency."

As it turned out, he had received a terrific job offer from the Keck School of Medicine, a part of the USC Norris Comprehensive Cancer Center, one of the finest teaching cancer hospitals in the world and a hotbed of leading-edge cancer research. We were very happy for him, but not so much for ourselves, as we had developed quite a strong bond with him.

"There are many fine doctors here at OHSU," he said, "and we can set up a program of yearly checkups for you."

"But what if I wanted to travel down to L.A. once a year?"

"That would be wonderful!" he said with a broad smile. "I would love to keep you as a patient."

And so began my annual trek down to the USC Norris Comprehensive Cancer Center, located in the Los Angeles area between Pasadena and San Gabriel.

Chapter Forty-Five

In the fall of 2009, I had invested in a small "boutique" speaker company that had been founded by a good friend over twenty years previously. They were seeing their business decline as the big-box retailers like Best Buy supplanted the neighborhood audio/video stores. They appointed me CEO, and we went about re-inventing the company as an online retailer.

I became a true Portlander. I sold my car, tuned up my old steel Trek hybrid bike, and outfitted it with fenders, lights, and flashers of all types. I rented a small office in Old Town Portland, bought a full-body cycling rain suit, and rode my bike the quick two miles to and from my office every day, rain or shine. All I lacked were multiple tats and some strategically placed piercings to become a real Portland bicycle commuter! I also got a new primary-care physician, and when I told her I had not felt depressed in a long time, she recommended that I stop taking the antidepressant. I discontinued it without incident and have not looked back.

On November 23rd, 2009, shortly after our move to Portland, I read a disturbing article in the local newspaper about Maurice Lucas. Lucas was the 6' 9" power forward for the Portland Trail Blazers' 1977 NBA championship team. Nicknamed "The Enforcer," he epitomized the tough, strong, tenacious style of play that took the team to the finals, eventually defeating the Philadelphia 76ers in one of the most exciting playoff series ever. So you can imagine my feelings when I read the headline that day: "Blazers Great Maurice Lucas Hospitalized; Bladder Cancer Has Returned."

The case of Maurice Lucas had special meaning for me, and not just because I had bladder cancer. Lucas was my age; he was born just a few months before me in 1952. He had complained of fatigue in late 2007 while working as an assistant coach for the Trail Blazers, right around the time of my diagnosis and the big decision on the surgery. In early 2008 he was diagnosed with T1 Grade III bladder cancer, exactly what I had. But he chose a different path, deciding against radical surgery and opting for the bladder-sparing regimen at a Portland hospital.

Tumors continued to show up throughout his treatments and he underwent several TURBTs. Eventually, in February 2009, his latest tumor was diagnosed as muscle invasive, and he underwent radical surgery on March 31st, 2009. Although the surgery was pronounced a success and he had announced plans to return to the team for the 2009-2010 NBA season, he was in the exact same place Dr. Daneshmand had so forcefully described to me. He had played defense.

So the headline on November 23rd hit me like a bag of bricks. His bladder cancer had metastasized at some point, and the surgery had not been able to get all of the cancer that had spread to his lymph nodes. Now it was back in force, and further surgery would be ineffective. Lucas spent weeks in the hospital undergoing chemotherapy, and eventually resigned his coaching position.

Maurice Lucas died at his home of metastatic bladder cancer on October 31st, 2010. He was fifty-eight years old.

Chapter Forty-Six

January 2011 was a major milestone in my cancer journey. I had learned that over 80% of bladder cancer recurrences following radical cystectomy (bladder removal) occur within the first three years. My ten-year survival chances went from under 50% to over 80%, and when I breezed through my tests at USC Norris Dr. Daneshmand estimated my chances to be even higher that that.

It was then that we started a practice that continues to this day; we ended the day with him interviewing me in detail about quality-of-life issues, including daytime and nighttime continence, potency, and mental and emotional health. I told him I considered my quality of life to be nothing short of amazing, all things considered. Then I asked him the purpose of the interviewing process. His response surprised me.

"At this point, Frank, you are teaching us," he said. "Every year that goes by, your experiences add to our understanding of the physical, mental, and emotional aspects of recovery from advanced bladder cancer. But I have one more question. Is there anything you regret about your treatment, before, during, or after your surgery?"

It was an easy question to answer, as I had thought about it for some time. "Absolutely no knock on you, because you were very thorough and 100% honest with me about everything before and after the cystectomy. The one thing I wish I had been able to do was talk to someone who had actually been through the surgery and had the neobladder. There were two aspects of the recovery, especially in the first two weeks, for which I was not at all prepared and, quite honestly, scared the shit out of me."

"And what were those two things?"

I told him the first was the incredible, unbelievable fatigue that I described earlier in this book. The second was the difficulty in recovering from the gastrointestinal part of the surgery. When thinking about the operation, one tends to naturally focus on the creation of the working neobladder as the urinary system, as it sounds like science fiction! The actual recovery from that part of the surgery is actually pretty straightforward. It's the removal of a meter of small intestine that just completely clobbers the entire digestive system, and I had really not taken that as seriously as I might have.

So he asked me if I would be willing to speak to male patients in my general age group who were either considering the neobladder route or already scheduled for it. I told him I would jump at the chance to help others.

I've found that there are two distinct types of post-cancer

folks. The first, and likely the most common, wants to forget the whole experience and not revisit it other than from a medical standpoint—regular checkups and the like. This person does not like to talk about cancer, especially their own, and often strongly requests that relatives and friends alike refrain from bringing it up, even in innocent conversations that come around to cancer. It's important to understand that this does not mean that they feel ashamed or guilty about their cancer, and it's certainly their decision to make.

The second type of person embraces the experience and is comfortable talking about cancer and even sharing the details of their own experiences with the disease. You can probably guess into which category a person who writes a book about his cancer experiences might fall.

Chapter Forty-Seven

One of the significant outcomes of that January visit was that I started viewing my body a bit differently. One day in late March 2011 I looked at myself in the bathroom mirror after my morning shower and realized I was looking at a potentially very unhealthy person. I was sporting love handles and a pretty fair start at man-boobs, neither of which I had ever had, in addition to a very large pot belly. My neck was thick and saggy with fat and my face was fuller and rounder than it had ever been. My old inner voice began to speak for the first time since my illness.

"Hey, stupid," it said, "you're fat and getting fatter. You made it to three years and you're probably not going to die. Don't kill yourself some other way just because you survived cancer."

Shaking my head, I dug in the back of the closet and found the old electronic scale I had used weekly in 2004, when I lost a lot of weight on the low-carb South Beach Diet. I dragged it into the bathroom, and hopped on.

I weighed 254 pounds.

I was stunned. I knew I was heavy, but at my worst I had never been close to 250, ever. Even when I did the diet in 2004 I started at 238 pounds, at the time the heaviest I had ever been. I resolved to start the South Beach Diet again as soon as possible. For various reasons, including my own inability to make the commitment I knew was absolutely necessary to get through the critical first two weeks (Phase One), I didn't finally start the diet until April 25, 2011.

It took thirty-five weeks, but I managed to lose fifty-six pounds and achieve my goal of a sustainable weight of under two hundred pounds. On December 19th, 2011, I climbed on the scale for the weekly Monday morning weigh-in. I weighed 198 pounds.

For the first three years following my surgery, I worked hard on improving my nighttime continence, which any neobladder owner/operator will tell you is among the biggest challenges. I had developed my own bedtime ritual, a series of deep breathing exercises and various stretching and relaxation techniques, interspersed with repeated urination. By this method, I was able to almost completely empty the neobladder. Over the years you develop a kind of sixth sense about fullness, even though you don't have the stretched-muscle feeling of a conventional full bladder. Through this nightly process, I was able to limit myself to a few drops escaping most nights and an "episode" of incontinence happening only about every three weeks.

Then a crazy thing happened to me, just as I was approaching my target weight on the diet. For some strange reason, perhaps the low-carb nature of the diet or perhaps just the weight loss itself, I became nighttime incontinent again. No matter how diligently I went through my nightly ritual, I could still sense that my bladder was not completely empty. Then, an hour or two after I went to sleep, my muscles would just involuntarily release, and I would flood the bed. I was wearing an adult absorbency product to bed, but even with that protection we were awake changing sheets almost every other night. You probably remember my earlier comments about the smell.

This continued for two weeks. I was extremely frustrated by this unexpected turn of events, and mortified that I was putting my wife through this after all the patient support she had provided for almost four years.

One night I was in the final stages of my relaxation ritual, and I was angry because I knew I was not empty. I pulled open the bottom drawer of the cabinet below our sinks. There was the travel kit that contained the catheter, lube, and irrigation solution. I stared at the catheter for a long time.

There is probably no one on this planet that dislikes catheterization more than I do, especially having had to perform it on myself, if only a few times back in the beginning of my recovery. I thought of my long-suffering wife lying a few feet away in bed and knew we would be up in an hour or two, and I was angry.

"It's the lesser of two evils, for sure," I thought to myself as I reached into the drawer.

As much as I dreaded it, the whole process took less than five minutes and was not painful at all. I felt a strange pride and sense of accomplishment as I cleaned the equipment carefully and headed to bed.

I slept for seven hours and awoke as dry as a bone. I've been catheterizing right before bed every night since, and my incontinence is a thing of the past. Of course, I contacted Dr. Daneshmand and told him about it, but he had always been very candid that many patients require nightly or even every-few-hours catheterization to stay continent. This time he told me it was absolutely fine, and would ensure that the neobladder was 100% empty once every twenty-four hours. This was actually very good for neobladder health, as it prevents mucous build-up that can foster infections.

FEAR

Chapter Forty-Eight

When my wife was diagnosed with cancer ten years ago, the first person I called was my dear friend whose wife had died from breast cancer. It was her tragic passing that got me started volunteering for the Lance Armstrong Foundation. I remember that conversation almost verbatim.

When I told him of Laura's diagnosis, he said, "Your life will never be the same from this day forward. Every day when you wake up you will think to yourself, 'Is today the day?' And one day I woke up and today was the day."

Since then I have had many conversations with him about my cancer journey. Not to minimize the seriousness of being the spouse and caregiver of a cancer patient, but when it's yourself you're talking about, the "Is today the day?" question becomes much more weighty.

Following another successful visit to USC Norris in January

2012, I was not thinking much about cancer. I had been completely cancer-free for over four years, and I was feeling quite healthy, particularly after the weight loss. So you can imagine my surprise when I awoke on the morning of Tuesday, April 10th, 2012.

When I went to the bathroom to drain my bladder, the first thing I saw was several small chunks of coagulated blood that looked almost black. This was unusual, but not a first. Dr. Daneshmand and I had discussed this as it had happened three or four times over the previous four years, usually following strenuous physical exertion or a long bike ride. He always cautioned me that any actual uncoagulated blood in the urine or mucous was the number one danger signal for a recurrence of bladder cancer, typically coming from metastases in the urethra or kidneys. I remembered him calling it "symptoms consistent with recurrence," a phrase that still gives me the chills.

When I was finished urinating, the whole bowl had an unmistakable light pink tinge, and the mucous was a dark pink color. Blood. For certain, 100%. The number one indicator of recurrence. Needless to say, I was completely freaked out. Terrified and angry that after four years plus, cancer-free, it was back. The words of my friend echoed in my head.

Was today the day?

By early afternoon, my urine was a darker pink and the small amount of mucous was a very dark pink, almost red. With shaking hands and dread in my heart I quickly composed an email to Dr. Daneshmand with a detailed description of each incident. I'm sure he could feel the desperate tone of my message. He replied that it was very likely nothing to panic about. His calm demeanor came through loud and clear. In my message, I had also mentioned that the night before I noticed the blood I had felt a slight twinge somewhere inside when I catheterized before bed. We theorized that I could have inadvertently "nicked" some of the internal tissue with the tip of the catheter, but blood is not something you ignore if you're a bladder cancer veteran.

He sent me off immediately to OHSU in Portland for blood and urine tests to see if there was any evidence of cancer cells. When those tests came back negative late that day, he advised me to wait and see if the blood increased or went away over the following forty-eight hours.

First morning urine on Wednesday the 11th was light yellow with no pink tinge and the mucous was its normal off-white color. I reported this to Dr. Daneshmand and he said there was no reason to rush down to California unless the bleeding started up again, but he wanted me to come down in a week or ten days for a battery of tests including ultrasound and a thorough cystoscopy.

Chapter Forty-Nine

I was blood-free for the next few days, so I booked a flight to Burbank for a week later. My confidence was permanently shaken, however, and my first thoughts every day were about cancer. Was today the day?

The week passed quickly and uneventfully, and on Wednesday, April 18th, I kissed my wife goodbye and headed for the Portland airport and my flight south. I checked into the same Hilton hotel in San Gabriel that I had stayed in just a few months back when I was down for my annual January tests. I remembered how confident and worry-free I had been, having just celebrated the four-year anniversary of The Big Cut. I was comforted in that I had seen no more evidence of bleeding, but my confidence had been badly shaken.

Early the next morning I ate a light breakfast and headed to USC Norris. It started like my regular routine, with blood work, urine sample, and chest x-ray, followed by ultrasound of the neobladder and kidneys. This was important, because bladder cancer almost never recurs inside the neobladder since it's not a real bladder, coming from a different part of the body, the digestive tract.

Following the long ultrasound session, I was taken to a different treatment room where Dr. Daneshmand waited with the cystoscope. A typical cystoscopy takes only a few minutes, but this one lasted over a half-hour, as he wanted to look carefully at every bit of my insides. I watched it all in color on a large high-definition, flat-panel monitor. It was fascinating to see the new bladder from the inside, as all of my previous tests had been cystograms, where I was being looked at from the outside.

The test concluded with the cystoscope being very slowly withdrawn a millimeter at a time so he could examine every bit of the urethra, from its juncture with the neobladder to the opening. Dr. Daneshmand had cautioned me that this might be pretty uncomfortable but was absolutely necessary. In fact, like most of these procedures, it sounds far worse than it actually was. For once, the "mild discomfort" moniker was accurate.

Throughout the day, Dr. Daneshmand was calm and reassuring, giving his opinion that he was not going to find anything, along with his reassurance that if he did we would deal with it. But knowing the statistics around mortality rates after recurrence—not good at all—I was extremely concerned.

The day concluded at around 3:00 p.m. with a final consultation in yet another examination room to review all the results. The twenty minutes waiting there were some of the longest of my life. When I saw the familiar smile on Dr. Daneshmand's face as he entered, I knew immediately that I had not suffered a recurrence. He started out with the cytology results, assuring me that the results were identical to those the previous week at OHSU: there was zero indication of cancer. Then he showed me stills of the ultrasound, which showed no abnormalities or masses in the kidneys.

Finally we moved on to the cystoscopy. He told me that he had seen absolutely nothing, not even any trace of scarring that might indicate that I had in fact nicked myself internally while catheterizing. He emphasized that this was still the most likely explanation and that the ten days that had elapsed was plenty of time for whatever damage had been done to heal. His last comment was the big one.

"Based on every test we did today," he said, "I can say with 100% certainty that you do not have recurring cancer."

I thanked him profusely with tears in my eyes. He said he understood my concern due to the seriousness of bladder cancer recurrence, but that he had been very confident that he wouldn't find anything, based on the detailed description of the symptoms that I had provided and the negative tests at OHSU the day of the bleeding incident. Of course, he also said that the follow-up tests were well worth it, if only for my own peace of mind.

Driving back to the Burbank airport, I knew that my life had changed, once again, forever. I would never again forget about cancer for weeks at a time as I had following my four-year all clear. I knew for sure I would think about recurrence every day going forward. I expected to feel euphoric after I called Laura with the good news and checked in for my flight—and in fact we did drink a very good bottle of wine later that evening in Portland—but even though I was awash with feelings of relief and gratitude, I didn't feel the unbounded joy I had expected to feel when I heard the results. I realized the simple truth. It was just another day, with many more to come. There was only one thing different.

Today was not the day.

Epilogue

L ance Armstrong was the first person I ever heard use the phrase, "the blessing of cancer." It was at a private meeting of the volunteer regional mentors that was held every year prior to the Ride for the Roses in Austin, and I was in my second year as the regional for the Pacific Northwest. It was 2004, and Lance had just won his sixth consecutive Tour de France in July. I remember thinking that it was an absurd statement. How could anyone look at cancer as a blessing?

Over the previous couple of years, I had seen my beautiful wife endure surgery and brutal chemotherapy, and had attended the funeral of one of my best friends' wife. I was not in a place to think about some kind of "blessing of cancer." But Lance continued.

"Of course," he said, "if there was any way I could have avoided it I would have. But it has made me a better person.

It has enabled me to focus my energies. I can tell you, for certain, that I would have never won a major stage race, ever, much less win the Tour six times, had I not had cancer."

As I write this in the fall of 2014, approaching the seventh anniversary of my surgery, I remember those words. Because now I, too, refer frequently to the blessing of cancer. Like anyone, I would never have chosen it, but I can honestly say that the last seven years have been by far the happiest of my life. I feel that I am a better husband, a better father, and a better friend than I ever would have been if cancer had not tried and failed to destroy my life.

Today I am in excellent health, and my overall quality of life is nothing short of miraculous considering the severity of my illness. I am fastidious about cleanliness, and have never once suffered the most common complication with a neobladder, a UTI (urinary tract infection). My digestive episodes have steadily declined in both frequency and intensity over the years. I needed no chemotherapy or radiation, and the only medication related to my cancer is a daily sublingual dose of vitamin B12, as the meter of small intestine that was relocated to build the neobladder is the section that normally absorbs that vitamin.

But, everything I just wrote above notwithstanding, I hate cancer. I hate it with every ounce of energy I have, and that hatred resides in every fiber of my being. Cancer hurt me. Bad. I would love to proclaim that I stand here today unbeaten and unbowed, but that would be a lie. Cancer mutilated me physically, mentally, and emotionally. It has made me largely ineffective in the sport of cycling, an activity that once defined me, not to mention my physical fitness. It drove me to consider myself a failure. It drove me to depression. It hurt me badly.

I continue to counsel men around my age who are facing either the decision about bladder cancer surgery or who are already scheduled for it. I have spoken with over a dozen patients from both OHSU and USC Norris. I try to calmly but honestly answer the usual questions without alarming them unnecessarily or sugarcoating the procedures. They all want to know about incontinence and impotence, of course, but I always try to answer the unasked questions as well. I tell them about the two things for which I was simply not prepared, the crushing fatigue and the digestive meltdowns.

At my last yearly check-up, I was telling Dr. Daneshmand how much I enjoyed counseling his patients prior to surgery, and had followed through with several for up to a year post-cystectomy. I was surprised to hear that based on my success with these patients, USC Norris has expanded the counseling by adding other "specialists," a younger man in his forties, an older man, and, yes, a woman who had a neobladder built by Dr. Daneshmand. This was really gratifying to me.

I am also a regular contributor to the Bladder Cancer Advocacy Network (BCAN), an online community for bladder cancer patients and caregivers. I typically post on the specific subjects I have spoken about in this book, whenever I feel that my experiences may add some value to the conversation. BCAN does a wonderful job of enabling the sharing of information and knowledge, and they deserve support.

Many people who have lived through the cancer experience have an intuitive idea of what caused their cancer. I am no exception. Bladder cancer is the second cancer scientifically proven to be caused by cigarette smoking, after lung cancer. The carcinogens are cleaned from the blood by the kidneys and passed down to the bladder, the mucous membranes of which are constantly bathed in carcinogens. Although I have never been a smoker, I worked for long periods in Europe, both with Amazon and with D&M Holdings, in the days before Europe became enlightened about smoking in restaurants and public spaces. I attended many business dinners where virtually everyone was smoking, and many trade show meetings where fifteen or twenty people were packed into a small, unventilated conference room, all smoking. I believe that second-hand smoke was to blame for my tumors.

I treasure my yearly visits with Dr. Daneshmand, whom I am honored to call a friend. He is the most compassionate and caring medical professional I have ever had the good fortune to meet. He updates me on the constant evolution of the surgery and on his team's focus on easier recovery and long-term quality of life. In fact, the recovery process today is far quicker and significantly easier that it was in 2007, thanks to the hard work and dedication of the team at USC Norris.

These days, when it comes to cancer, I have chosen to replace the darkness of hatred with the promise of discovery and progress. Allow me to explain.

In January of this year, following my day of tests, I was having dinner at the L.A. Prime Steakhouse at the top of the Westin Bonaventure Hotel in downtown Los Angeles with Dr. Daneshmand and John Baker, senior executive director in the fundraising and philanthropy division at USC Norris. He is also a rabid basketball fan, and the three of us were headed to the L.A. Lakers game after our dinner.

Our conversation was around treatments for cancer. We were bemoaning the sad fact that little has really changed in the last hundred years. Sure, the surgeries are safer and more effective, as are the chemo and radiation regimens. But the truth is that all we really know how to do to treat this disease is cut, poison, and burn. Same as it ever was. I mentioned a lecture I had been to at OHSU given by Dr. Brian Drucker, the inventor of a whole new type of cancer treatment based on genetics and immunotherapy. He discovered the genetic cause of a type of leukemia (chronic myeloid leukemia) and developed a drug called Gleevec, approved in 2001, which effectively cures it with a pill a day.

Since then, this genetic approach with immunotherapy has been successfully tested in clinical trials for metastasized melanoma (skin cancer) and a few other cancers. I asked Dr. Daneshmand if this approach might be relevant in bladder cancer treatment. He said it certainly was, but that there was little or no funding for the necessary research. He went on to say that his research team had actually outlined a project and that they were already freezing tissue samples in case funding became available.

That dinner conversation led to further discussion among Dr. Daneshmand, John Baker, and Laura and me, and culminated in June with our agreeing to personally fund the project over the next two years. It is now underway with promising preliminary results, and represents one of the first-ever such research projects in the bladder cancer arena.

We are excited and proud to be a part of this leading-edge research, and with the dedication and expertise of Dr. Daneshmand and his team we are confident that many other bladder cancer patients will make the journey back to life.

Portland, Oregon
November 2014

Acknowledgements

When I began working on this book in early 2014, I had no idea what an emotional roller coaster ride I was starting. Reliving the story day by day put me through a wringer in ways I had not imagined. I always expected that the sections about making the decision and the surgery and early recovery would be gut-wrenching for me, but it became much more than that. Writing about the loss of friends, my depression following the 2008 Ride for the Roses fail, and even recounting the amazing act of camaraderie and compassion showed by the two Yellow Jersey riders near the end of the ride that day, all affected me deeply.

As the book developed, it became clear to me that although this memoir will certainly find some interest in the bladder cancer community, it was not really written for bladder cancer patients, or even cancer survivors in general.

Rather, it is aimed at anyone who wants to follow an unexpected adventure from the point of view of the reluctant adventurer.

However, as mentioned way back in chapter thirty, I am more than willing to discuss even the most intimate and clinical details with any cancer patient or caregiver. My counsel should be especially relevant to anyone who is in the process of making a decision on treatment for bladder cancer, particularly neobladder surgery. Speaking with someone who has been through the decision-making process, not to mention the surgery itself, is likely to be valuable to most patients. Feel free to contact me at any time at frank@bladdercancerjourney.com and we can set up a time to talk by phone.

I know there are many errors in this final manuscript, particularly in the medical arena. All of them are mine alone. For example, the survival percentage for T3 Grade III bladder cancer is considerably higher than the 5% I cite in chapter three. I considered correcting this but decided against it. Even though I have been unable to locate the Web site where I first saw that number, I am quite certain that I did see it, and my reaction to it as described in that chapter was terrifying and genuine.

I mentioned in chapter eighteen that many of my memories are suspect, particularly in the two-week period right after the surgery. There are other examples. In reading my account of returning to the Ride for the Roses in October 2008, I recalled telling Lance Armstrong that I missed the 2007 ride due to cancer. That conversation happened as reported. But, as my brilliant and long-suffering editor, Mary

Anne Ericson, has pointed out, the initial episode of bleeding did not occur until the week after the 2007 ride. Further research revealed that I had decided in August not to attend due to my new company's annual planning meeting in Yokohama, Japan, which took place the same week as the ride.

My sincere thanks go out to the aforementioned Mary Anne Ericson, who assumed the dual role of both content and copy editor. She does great work, and her patience and skill are largely responsible for whatever positive attributes this final manuscript may possess. She is one of the smartest people I have ever had the pleasure to know, and it was an honor to work with her.

Special thanks to all of my friends who have suffered my incessant babbling about every aspect of this endeavor for the past ten months, including, but certainly not limited to, Pete Sommerfeld, Joel Scotchler, Meg Thomas, John Healey, Jeri Beck, Brad and Patti Beegle, Don and April Brenneman, Patrick Zahn, Jason Sather, Dave Pendleton, and Dorinda Van Dusen. Extra special thanks to Kirk Sewell, bartender extraordinaire, who put up with my cancer-book chatter at least three nights a week throughout the writing and editing process.

Several of my colleagues from the consumer electronics industry were instrumental in getting me through my cancer experience: Roland MacBeth, Greg Keys, Kevin Weinhoeft, Norman Olson, Karl Bearnarth, Jim Minarik, and Murray Huppin, to name just a few. They are giants.

An individual shout-out must certainly go to my friend Jeff Smith and his wife Cheryl. With his frequent visits, hilarious get-well cards, and fancy water, he kept me upbeat in some of my darkest hours. He also got me back on my bike more than once. Thank you, Jeff.

I have been blessed with a wonderful family. Thanks to my three marvelous children, all adults now. Keith, Alison, and Craig, along with Keith's lovely wife Katie, gave me unconditional support and love, without which my journey would have been infinitely more difficult.

Dr. Sia Daneshmand and his incredible teams, both at OHSU here in Portland and now at USC Norris in Los Angeles, unquestionably saved my life, no matter what their modesty may compel them to claim. It is because of them that I have seen my children grow into adults, celebrated birthdays into my sixties, and held two granddaughters in my arms. It is impossible to thank them enough.

Lastly, this book is dedicated to my wife Laura Ann Sadowski. She cared for me with tenderness, love, and good humor through situations that were not fair for her to have to endure. She is the best person I have ever known. Thank you, Laura.

About the Author

FRANK SADOWSKI was an English and journalism major at the University of Delaware, and served as the features editor of the university's newspaper, the *Review*, for two years. He has worked in the consumer electronics industry in many different capacities for over forty years, and currently is self-employed as a business consultant specializing in e-commerce. This is his first book. He also pens a highly entertaining, eclectic blog, *Frank-Incensed*, at fsadowski.blogspot.com. He is an avid cyclist, which figures large in *Back to Life*. He lives with his wife Laura in Portland, Oregon, and Las Vegas, Nevada.

Please visit www.bladdercancerjourney.com to view a gallery of original photographs depicting the actual events in this book. There you can also post your comments, inquire about author readings and book signings, and even book a live Skype session with the author for your book club.

Made in the USA
Las Vegas, NV
18 November 2022

59734611R00120